Building Your Healthy Family

Balancing Nutrition, Movement and Time

Kathy Tonelli

ISBN:1717521215
ISBN-13: 978-1717521217

Cover photos by Alex Terreault

Printed in the United States of America

I dedicate this book to my parents and first teachers, Richard and Nancy Kollet. They gave me the healthy start that I needed to become the person that I am today. They taught me the value of good food, an active lifestyle and managing time wisely.

CONTENTS

INTRODUCTION

We all want a healthy family. Take a minute and visualize a healthy family. What do its members look like and do? How do they think and act? What do they put into their bodies? What are their daily habits and rituals? How do they feel? What do they project to the world?

Each of us will visualize a different family and "see" different images as we contemplate each of the questions above. Maybe we are visualizing our own family or a fictional family. In either case, the images we "see" probably depict people who are healthy in weight, put good healthy foods into their bodies, have a "glow" about them and think positively about themselves. They are probably active and participate in healthy habits and rituals, such as exercising regularly, getting good sleep and taking care of their body's needs. These people most likely look healthy and happy and project a vigor for life to the world.

That can be every family. It takes effort. It takes work. Every family will have a different starting point, but we can all have the same destination. Some will have far to go and some not far at all.

The health of families has changed over the past few decades. There are very few people who mirror your visualization. Do you know anyone who measures up to what you "saw" in that healthy family? In reality, a large percentage of people are overweight, tired, stressed and generally feel like they are running on empty a lot of the time. This general change in health status has been driven, in part, by changes in ideas about what constitutes healthy and unhealthy foods, the increase in fast food options and the increase in convenience foods. These are foods that are processed and packaged. They are heavy on preservatives, sugars, fats and empty calories. It has also been driven by the fast paced, overscheduled lifestyle that many people live. A lifestyle that leaves little time for eating well and taking care of our bodies' needs for exercise, social interactions, relaxation, spiritual practices and sleep.

I grew up in the 1970s and 80s. I was raised in a fairly healthy household where we ate from-scratch meals the majority of the time. My brother and I played outside a lot riding our bikes, climbing trees, building forts, exploring the woods and playing whiffle ball and Hide and Seek with the neighborhood children. I was a Girl Scout and took swim lessons at a local pool. That was about all that was offered for kids in the small town where I grew up. Throughout my early years I was sheltered from many of the new fads in food.

Then along came the 80s and fast food options were increasing by the day. My little town now had, not one, but two, popular fast food burger restaurants. Packaged food choices took over the grocery store shelves. Cereal took up an entire aisle! Cookies and crackers had their own aisle, too. It was also in the 80s that fat became known as the big no-no. The waistlines of the general population were expanding rapidly and it was thought that eating fat made you fat. So, in came low-fat, no fat varieties of every packaged food under the sun! Grocery shelves now included all of these new "healthier" foods. Freezer sections were sporting as many options as the other aisles. The choices were endless! Why would you cook when you could buy all your meals in a box?

The American public was faced with such a myriad of choices and information they didn't know what to do. Most went along with the new healthier, low or no fat foods thinking they were doing themselves and their families a favor. What was really happening was far worse than anyone imagined. Fat adds flavor to foods. When the fat is removed, foods lose their original appeal. Sugar and artificial flavors are then added to give the food back its flavor. Back in the eighties this led to people consuming large amounts of sugars and artificial ingredients and preservatives. We now know that these carbohydrates and artificial additives cause not only obesity, but numerous chronic health issues.

As our diets got less and less healthy, life was getting busier and busier. There were more and more households where both parents worked. The 80s were a time of prosperity for many Americans and with two adults working they were able to have the latest gadgets, go on fancy vacations and buy larger homes. These families benefitted greatly from the well-stocked grocery shelves and freezers. Meals could be prepared and eaten quickly. There was no time to cook a meal between work and getting family members to the many activities they were involved in and enjoyed.

Stress levels increased because of the fast-pace that life had taken on. Getting everyone up and out in the morning and home and to bed at the end of the day was challenging. There was limited time for activities that promoted relaxation. When there was time available, the average family sat in front of the television and watched the endless string of sit-coms that were popular at the time.

This was the beginning of the era of innumerable choices of convenience foods, whether purchased at the local grocery store or from the local fast food restaurant. Americans began to set themselves up for the chronic health issues that arose and continue to plague large numbers of people today.

Today I am passionate about helping others get healthy. For years I watched as my mother struggled with weight issues. As a registered nurse, she listened to the recommendations of the time and went with the low-fat, no-fat options of many of the foods available, which didn't solve her weight problems. Over time, our family got busier, and she, too, fell prey to the packaged convenience foods for our snacks or for nights when our schedules were too demanding to make a real meal.

In 1989, I graduated from college and became an elementary school teacher. For the past three decades I have watched as more and more children have become overweight. I have watched their snacks become more processed and artificial. Each new "generation" of processed food seems less healthy, but more child centered. In came blue yogurt and rainbow gummies! School lunches became less healthy and lunches brought from home were a bunch of little pre-packaged, kid-sized containers of processed foods. I have watched kids become more sluggish and less energetic. Outdoor, unstructured playtime for the average child has practically vanished, but screen time has increased exponentially! The general core strength in children has decreased dramatically over the years. Many children can no longer comfortably sit upright on the floor or at their desk for more than a few minutes. They don't display the stamina or desire to participate fully in classroom activities. The average classroom is far too slow paced for them. Today's children have had fast paced, electronic toys and games from the time they were born. Their afterschool hours are full of extracurricular programs and activities. Children regularly say things like, "I don't have time to do this homework." "I won't have time to do my twenty minutes of reading. I have a hockey game tonight." "I'm so tired because I didn't get to bed until 10:00 last night because I had football practice and then I had to have a shower." Many children are overprogrammed, sleep deprived and feeling stressed and anxious. Parents are often encouraging them to participate in more activities and often make excuses for their children regarding homework and absences from school. Sadly, many of the parents I see are mirrors of their offspring. They are overweight, exhausted, running from one thing to the next and stressed.

My children, now in their early adult years, grew up during this latter time period and my family was not immune to the many commodities out there. My children ate their fair share of packaged foods, had electronic toys and video game systems and participated in scouts and played on local sports teams.

I worried about some of the choices we made and tried to find a balance, keeping their health in mind, yet not wanting them to feel deprived of the things their friends did and had.

There came a point when they were young teenagers that I began to consciously make food and lifestyle changes for our family that were healthier in nature. While dealing with chronic Lyme Disease myself I began doing a lot of research on natural ways to improve my own health. By making drastic lifestyle changes including changing many of the foods we purchased and the products we used, cutting back on our social schedule, and taking better care of our needs for exercise, stress reduction and sleep, I was able to regain my own health and set my family on a better path for lifelong health.

Realizing the positive impact of living a healthy, well balanced lifestyle I became certified as an integrative nutrition health coach in order to take my passion for health and wellness to the next step. I am now able to guide and support others in making healthy lifestyle changes for themselves and their families. Change is hard, but it's possible. This book is intended to guide parents and caregivers in making the long-lasting lifestyle changes necessary for their family to become healthier in body, mind and spirit. Think now about your own family's starting point as you ready yourself for the journey you are about to embark on toward lifelong health and wellness.

Chapter One

Feeding Your Family

Food is the mainstay of our existence. Without it we cannot survive. It is what nourishes our bodies and keeps us alive. It can make us healthy or it can make us sick. In this modern era, much of what we consume is a combination of processed food byproducts, natural and artificial colorings and flavorings, chemical additives, and preservatives that give many "foods" a shelf life of months to years. Many of our meals come from packages that we heat in a microwave or are prepared somewhere else to be eaten out or brought home. These, too, often come from a package. These processed "foods" do not provide good nourishment and keep us healthy. That being said, it is possible in this modern world to feed your family a healthy, well balanced diet.

With some basic knowledge, a few strategies and a little effort you can easily prepare healthy meals and snacks for your family. You may be thinking that you don't have time, you don't know much about healthy food, you don't know how to cook or that it's going to cost a lot of money. You are not alone if you are thinking some of these thoughts. Whenever we venture into something new, fears and doubts surface. Let's take a few minutes to explore these perceptions in a very basic sense. They will come up again in more detail in later chapters.

In any busy family, time is always of the essence. There is more time available in some families than in others, depending on personal schedules, however, with a little planning and practice, good, healthy meals can come together pretty quickly. Many simple, family friendly meals can be prepared in a half hour or less, with some needing additional cooking time. If you typically get a lot of your meals and snacks out, you will probably find that it is often less time consuming and almost as convenient to prepare and eat foods at home. It takes time to drive to and from a restaurant, order food, wait for it to be served and eat. When you cook and eat at home, you are in control and can plan accordingly based on the day's schedule. If the meal needs to bake or simmer for a bit, you can be accomplishing other things while it cooks. You may even find you gain some additional time once you get this new habit established.

Let's look at some food basics. First and foremost, real, whole (or minimally processed) foods are the building blocks of a healthy diet. What are real, whole foods? These are foods that are recognizable. They are foods your grandmother and even your great grandmother, if she were alive today, would recognize. These are fruits and vegetables, meats and fish, beans, eggs, whole grains, rice and oats, nuts and seeds. They are, for the most part, single ingredient foods. Healthy, whole grain breads are the exception and have about five natural ingredients. Real whole foods generally do not come in boxes or sealed in plastic bags. You may choose to include some minimally processed foods in your family's diet. If you do, follow these two rules of thumb to guide you in knowing what to purchase and what to leave behind. The first is a short ingredient list. Five ingredients or less is ideal, however, a few more, as will sometimes be found in trail mixes, for example, can be okay. The second rule of thumb, especially as the amount of ingredients increase, is that you have to be able to easily recognize each ingredient. If you come to words you don't recognize or can't pronounce, it doesn't qualify as a minimally processed food. Those words you don't recognize or can't say are most likely processed additives or preservatives. The bottom line is that good health is dependent on real, whole foods and ingredients. If you focus on foods that fit this description when shopping and preparing food you can feel confident that you are supporting the health of your family.

When it comes to making healthy meals, you don't have to have a lot of cooking experience or knowledge. Real, whole foods can be prepared simply and offer lots of flavor. Most kids prefer things on the simpler side anyway. They tend not to enjoy sauces and foods mixed together as much as adults. As long as you have the basic kitchen utensils, a cutting board and some cookware including a large fry pan, two or three saucepans of various sizes for use on the stovetop, a casserole dish or two and a cookie sheet or baking stone you'll be all set. You may need to follow some actual recipes to get started if you're looking for specific flavors. You can get simple recipes for any dish online, or you can buy a cookbook that focuses on simple meals from real, whole foods. Once you start cooking, you'll find the methods and flavors that work well for you and your family and preparing healthy meals and snacks will become second nature.

A common misconception is that buying real, whole food and ingredients is going to cost a lot of money. Many of the foods you will be buying are priced by the pound rather than the package. Sometimes prices may seem exorbitant, especially when you are purchasing fish, meats and out of season produce, but if you are used to purchasing take-out food or eating at restaurants, I think you'll be in for a pleasant surprise. Think about the average cost to feed your family a meal prepared out of the home. A take-out dinner for four costs between thirty and forty dollars. To eat dinner at a sit-down family restaurant it will cost the same family between eighty and hundred dollars. That is for one meal. The average person consumes twenty-one meals in a week. Five take out dinners for four at thirty-five dollars apiece would cost one hundred seventy-five dollars and two dinners at a sit-down restaurant for the same family at ninety dollars each would cost an additional one hundred eighty dollars. Altogether it would cost this family three hundred fifty-five dollars for one week's worth of dinners. Keep in mind breakfast, lunch and snacks haven't been accounted for. Even if you bought top quality foods at the grocery store, you could buy all the food to feed a family of four for a week for the cost of the seven dinners out. Most likely the grocery bill would be considerably less. The same is true if you typically purchase a lot of prepared, packaged meals and snacks. They can be quite costly. Also keep in mind that you usually have no idea of the quality of the ingredients in the food you consume when it is prepared at a restaurant or comes from a package. Typically, food businesses purchase in bulk and are likely less interested in quality than in price. Chances are you are spending a lot of money on low quality food. In reality, you can prepare delicious meals and snacks that your family will enjoy from higher quality foods for much less money.

Making the change to feeding your family a diet of real, whole foods prepared at home has many advantages and health benefits. With some planning and a bit of effort you can easily prepare healthy meals and snacks for your family.

Chapter Two

Planning Healthy Meals and Snacks

Your first step is to look at your family's schedule. I would start with one week, but you may choose to do it by the month. I advise you to take a few minutes to actually write this out. You will most likely just do this as you are getting started, though you may prefer to continue this on a weekly or monthly basis. Write it on a piece of paper or on a blank calendar. If you don't have a blank calendar around, you can easily make your own or find one on the internet. Many word processing programs contain printable calendars. If you prefer technology, do this activity right on your computer.

Now look at the schedule. What time does everyone need to be up and out in the morning? How much time is available? Will time allow for a cooked breakfast or will family members need to eat quickly or take something with them. Where is everyone at lunchtime? Will lunches need to be prepared to go? What activities take place after school, work and in the evening? On what days do they occur? Determine which days during the week all or some of your family is home for breakfast, lunch and dinner. How much time is available for meal prep and eating on those days? Are there some days you won't have time to prepare a fresh meal? Answering all of these questions will help guide you in planning what and how much to buy to make healthy meals for your family. This may seem tedious, but keep in mind that establishing new rituals and routines takes some work. Before long this will be second nature. It is likely that your family's general schedule will stay fairly consistent, so once you've gotten into the habit of thinking this way, it will take minimal effort.

Before heading to the store, use your family's schedule and your answers to the questions on the previous page to guide you in planning your meals for the week. When planning healthy meals and snacks there are a couple of things to keep in mind. There is more to putting together a healthy meal than just serving real, whole foods. First, all foods fall into one or more of three main categories. These categories are fats, proteins and carbohydrates. Here's a brief, surface level education on these. Fats, proteins and carbohydrates are known as the macronutrients. The term macro means large. The macronutrients are the nutrients that we need in large amounts to survive. A truly healthy meal (or snack) includes fat, carbohydrates and protein. As you begin planning healthy meals you may find this challenging. Don't worry! Before long you will know what foods fall into each category. For quick reference, use this chart of commonly agreed upon, whole foods listed by macronutrient category as you get started.

Macronutrient Category Chart

Fats	Carbohydrates	Proteins
Full fat, organic dairy - milk, cheese, yogurt and butter	Whole grains - rice, oats, barley and quinoa	Greek yogurt and milk
Nuts and nut butters	Fruits	Grass-fed and/or free-range organic meats

Fats continued	Carbohydrates continued	Proteins continued
Eggs and grass-fed beef	Vegetables	Wild caught salmon and other fish
Fatty fish - salmon, trout, sardines and herring	Whole grain breads	Beans and lentils
Avocados and coconut	Whole grain pastas	Eggs
Dark chocolate	Beans, peas and lentils	Nuts, nut butters and seeds
Extra virgin olive oil, coconut oil	Starchy vegetables - potatoes, sweet potatoes, corn	Leafy greens and cruciferous vegetables like broccoli

At this point you may be wondering what a balanced, healthy meal that includes foods from all three macronutrient categories looks like. In June of 2011, the United States Department of Agriculture replaced the old food pyramid with a new visual to help people balance the foods they put on their plates. According to this visual, half of your plate should be fruits and vegetables, with the goal of slightly more vegetables than fruits. The other half should be whole grain foods and protein with whole grains taking up more space than protein. They also recommend a small serving of dairy. To see the actual visual, search "choose my plate" in any search engine to locate the website. If you use this idea as your basic guide and serve real, whole foods, your family will be eating healthy meals. Depending on the meal, amounts in each section of the plate will vary some. If you are serving something like tacos, pizza or a casserole where foods will be mixed, be sure to include all three macronutrient groups. Go heavier on the fruits and/or vegetables and lighter on the protein when preparing dishes like this. Keep your carbs to about one third or less of the dish.

Here are some examples of balanced breakfasts, lunches, dinners and snacks to help guide you. Balanced, healthy snacks should also have a combination of fat, protein and carbohydrates, just like any meal.

Breakfasts

Oatmeal (from whole grain oats), made with milk (or a healthy milk alternative such as pure coconut milk), topped with fresh or frozen berries. You could add additional toppings like shredded coconut, granola, raisins or dried cranberries, chopped nuts, chia seeds, ground flaxseeds, sliced bananas or other fruits. You can take this to go, just take the toppings in a separate container and add after reheating.

An egg (any way you like it) with roasted, seasoned potatoes or a slice of whole grain toast, with fresh fruit.

Greek yogurt with fresh fruit, and any of the additional toppings listed with the oatmeal. Plain yogurt is healthiest, but don't worry about a flavored yogurt if that's what your family will eat. A healthier option is to buy a tub of flavored and a tub of plain and mix them 50/50. Once you add the extras, no one will know it's a mixture of the two. Yogurt also works well for on the go breakfasts. Again, add the toppings when you are ready to eat.

A sliced banana or sliced apple with peanut or almond butter makes a great breakfast for kids. You can sprinkle with some raisins or sunflower seeds for added nutrition. Sunflower seed butter is a nut free option.

Lunches

A sandwich of whole grain bread (whole grain, white breads are available for children who won't eat the other varieties), a filling such as tuna, egg or chicken salad, fresh turkey or chicken breast, topped with any of the following; lettuce, fresh spinach, fresh arugula, tomatoes, sliced onions, cucumbers or avocado. You can add a small amount of mustard or mayonnaise. Pair this with a piece of fruit or a cup of soup and you should have plenty of energy for the afternoon.

A fresh tossed, green salad topped with some kind of protein (meat, fish, beans, hummus, quinoa etc.). Feel free to add nuts, seeds, fruits (avocado is a fruit and is great on salad) and/or any roasted or fresh vegetables you have available. The possibilities are endless! Top with a healthy salad dressing. For a quick and easy homemade dressing combine two to three parts extra virgin olive oil with one part balsamic or apple cider vinegar. Add any herbs you like. (Don't be shy with the herbs. If you don't add enough you won't have good flavor. If you are using fresh herbs you'll need to increase amounts.) Shake your dressing to combine and enjoy. This dressing doesn't need to be refrigerated.

Leftovers from dinner also make a great lunch. You could supplement with a small salad if there's not quite enough.

For school lunches pack sandwiches on whole grain breads with kid friendly fillings. Pair with any of the following: fresh fruit (whole or cut up), cut up vegetables and "dip" (hummus, a healthy ranch dressing or guacamole), Greek yogurt with a small container or baggie of mix-ins such as fresh diced fruit or berries, granola or shredded coconut. Another kid friendly option is whole grain crackers to eat alone or to dip. Be creative.

Dinners

Grilled or baked meat (chicken, pork or beef), roasted potatoes, another vegetable of your choice (steamed broccoli, green beans or pea pods/grilled asparagus/roasted winter squash or carrots) and a tossed green salad with a healthy store bought or homemade dressing.

Fresh fish (grilled or baked), coleslaw, baked potatoes with real butter, ghee or sour cream.

Homemade pizza on whole grain crust with tomato sauce, a variety of cheeses (mozzarella, fresh grated parmesan and cheddar work well), toppings of your choice. Serve with a tossed salad, vegetables (carrots, grape tomatoes, cucumber spears, broccoli, cauliflower, celery, zucchini spears) and dip, a fresh fruit salad or fruit kabobs.

Beef or chicken stew, a tossed salad and a hearty, whole grain bread with real butter or ghee.

Snacks

Whole grain crackers and cheese.
Hummus and vegetables.
An apple, a banana or celery topped with peanut butter. Add raisins or sunflower seeds for added nutrients.
A half cup of whole milk Greek yogurt with any of the following: fresh or frozen berries, other chopped fruits, shredded coconut, ground flax seed, chia seeds or chopped nuts.

To avoid having to make several trips to the store, you'll want to plan your meals ahead of time and have ingredients on hand to prepare many different meals. You should also have an idea of what your family will have for snacks. Depending on what your current eating habits are and what you already have on hand, you may feel like you have to buy an excessive amount of food in order to prepare the meals you plan. You may need to buy seasonings and spices, oils and vinegars, sauces and broths. Don't worry, you don't use the entire container or package of everything you buy in a week, especially ingredients that are used in small amounts.

In addition to purchasing the ingredients you need for the meals you have planned for the week, you will want to start to build a supply of non-perishable items such as rice, pasta and beans, frozen fruits and vegetables, canned or jarred items and seasonings. These are typically called pantry items. Having basic items on hand that you use frequently will help you put meals together quickly if needed. Having a stocked pantry comes in handy when you are exceptionally busy and don't have time to plan the week's meals, or when plans change unexpectedly. If you end up working late or find you are having friends for dinner, you'll be able to put a healthy meal together right from your pantry. A well-stocked pantry includes a good variety of foods. You probably already have some of the recommended pantry items. You don't have to stock your pantry all at once. Pick up a few items each week and before long you'll be fully stocked with lots of healthy, non-perishables and frozen ingredients to use as needed. You'll find your pantry is a life saver! (See sample Pantry List on pages 12 and 13.)

Most meals and snacks made from real, whole foods will also contain at least some fresh items that you will have to buy more frequently. These will typically be the foods you refrigerate like meat, dairy and some fruits and vegetables, or the foods you store at room temperature like potatoes, onions and bananas. I've provided a general list to get you started. (See sample Fresh Foods List on page 13.)

Your actual meal plan will be based around what your family likes and will be your best guide for what to buy each week. Use the meal suggestions and food lists in this chapter as a guide for foods to include in your meals and snacks as you get started. I suggest you write out your menu for the week either on a calendar or a piece of paper. I personally use a dry erase board where I write the dinner menu each week. You may also want to add breakfasts and lunches right now, or at least ideas for those meals even if they are not assigned to a specific day. That way you won't leave any ingredients you need off your shopping list. When planning your menu start with simple meals. If you need a recipe search for one that is easy and has just a few ingredients. In addition, think about whether you could use leftovers from one meal to make part of another meal, or whether they could be made into lunches? For example, if you roast a chicken one night, you could use what is left to make a chicken soup, chicken sandwiches or a barbecue chicken pizza depending on how much chicken is left. If you plan to roast a chicken, you might want to purchase a slightly larger one, so you can use it for more than one meal. Something else to think about when planning your menu is whether you want to make a large batch of something to serve again on a busy night when there won't be much time for meal preparation or eating. Some meals are easy to make in large amounts and reheat easily and quickly. A few examples are meatballs and sauce, lasagna, soups and tuna/chicken/egg salad. Having leftovers to use again or add to lunches can save quite bit of time. Remember to keep your family's likes and dislikes in mind as you plan your meals and snacks and you'll be fine.

Pantry List

Dry Goods	Whole Grain Rice, Beans, Quinoa, Lentils, Pasta, Bread Crumbs, Oatmeal, Egg Noodles, Shredded Coconut, Dark Chocolate Bars, Semi-Sweet or Dark Chocolate Chips, Unbleached Regular and Whole Grain Flours, Sugar (regular unbleached cane sugar and brown sugar), Baking Powder, Baking Soda, Corn Starch, Cornmeal
Canned and Jarred Items	Peanut Butter and other Nut Butters, Real Fruit Jams, Nuts, Seeds, Canned Fish, Canned Beans, Jarred Tomato Products, Broths and Stocks (Vegetable, Chicken and/or Beef) Mustards, Mayonnaise, Olive Oil, Coconut Oil, Ghee, Vinegars, Cooking Wine, Ketchup, Soy Sauce or Coconut Amino, Pure Maple Syrup, Pure Unheated Local Honey, Salad Dressings, Applesauce, Pure Vanilla Extract, Whole Kernel Popcorn (for popping), Crackers
Frozen	Whole Grain Breads, Whole Grain English Muffins, Whole Grain Tortillas, Bagels, Frozen Vegetables (Corn, Peas, Carrots, Broccoli, Mixed (for stir fries, soups etc.)) Frozen Fruits (Blueberries, Strawberries, Mixed Berries), Meats (Chicken, Ground Beef/Turkey/Chicken), Fish, Cheese, Butter

Spices	Cinnamon, Nutmeg, Cloves, Allspice
Seasonings	Sea Salt, Pepper, Garlic Powder, Onion Powder, Parsley, Dill, Oregano, Basil, Paprika, Chili Powder, Crushed Red Pepper, Sage

Fresh Foods List

Buy Weekly	Buy Every Two to Three Weeks
Milk, Fruit Juice (NOT from Concentrate), Delicate Fruits (Fresh Berries, Grapes, Kiwi, Pre-Cut Fruits), Bananas, Salad Greens, Tomatoes, Cucumbers, Avocados, Peppers, Mushrooms, Fresh Herbs (Cut), Meats, Fish,	Yogurt, Citrus Fruits, Apples, Potatoes, Onions, Fresh or Jarred Garlic, Celery, Cabbage, Broccoli, Carrots, Cheese, Hummus, Eggs, Fresh Herbs (Potted)

You may be feeling overwhelmed right now, especially if you aren't in the habit of meal planning and cooking at home very often. You don't have to implement all of these ideas right away. Begin slowly and build up overtime. Plan to start with a couple of new meal ideas the first week. Purchase the ingredients needed for those particular meals along with some healthier snack foods as well as other items that your family is used to eating. This may be easier if you have older children who tend to be more set in their ways regarding food choices. On the other hand, you may decide to just go for it and make the change all at once. You know your family best. Either way, once you start planning your menu and preparing healthy food at home regularly, it will quickly become part of what you do and will require much less focused effort. Invite other family members to take part in the meal planning. Many kids get excited when they can plan a meal. Keep in mind this is a big change and change takes time. Don't be afraid to be creative and have fun with this!

Chapter Three

Shopping Strategies

Once you've got a menu planned for the week it's time to figure out just what you need to buy at the store. It's best to write a store list. You can jot it down on a piece of paper or put it into your smart phone. If you like to use technology you can search your app store for grocery shopping apps. Many will save your list so that you don't have to start from scratch every week. Some are color coded by food category. If you like that kind of thing, check them out. The important thing is that you find and use a method that works for you.

Give yourself plenty of time. Don't wait until you are ready to leave for the store. Find a time when the house is quiet and you can focus without being interrupted. Put your menu somewhere where you can see it. Go through each meal and write down what you need as you go. If you need more than one of an item, list how many you will need. Remember to list things like seasonings or condiments that you'll need to prepare or serve with the meal. A complete shopping list will save you extra trips to the store later in the week.

Once you've got your list made you're almost ready to go buy food, but before heading to the store there are a few things you should know regarding food quality and purchasing options. It is likely that you will be buying more fresh food items since a healthy diet consists primarily of meals made from real, whole foods. It is important to know that not all fresh foods are equal in quality. What is sold as fresh produce at your grocery store is probably not that fresh. It has most likely been shipped to the store on a truck and was harvested anywhere from several days to several weeks ago. It may have undergone many temperature changes and been treated with products designed to help food travel better and to preserve freshness. Fruits and vegetables are often picked too early, so they don't spoil during shipping or before they can be purchased. Be aware that fresh produce offers the best nutrition when picked at peak ripeness and when eaten as close to harvest as possible. Fruits and vegetables begin to lose nutrient value within hours of being picked.

When considering your source for fresh meats and fish the same ideas apply. If they were not locally sourced, how old are they? Where did they originate and how were they shipped? Have they been previously frozen? If so, then you cannot refreeze them before cooking.

There are two general rules of thumb to keep in mind when shopping for food. The first is to buy the highest quality you can afford and the second is that, generally speaking, the fresher the food, the better it is for you.

There are many places to purchase fresh foods other than your local grocery store. Depending on where you live and the time of year, your options will vary. You may be surprised what is available locally. Farmers' markets have popped up all over the place. Many are now open year-round and offer lots of fresh selections. Local farm stores are often open year-round, also. These markets and local farmers may not always have fresh produce available, but you can find eggs, honey, maple syrup, homemade preserves and baked goods, breads, meats and cheeses. Many farmers grow greens and other produce in greenhouses during the colder months and you can often find root vegetables, winter squashes, apples and apple products available throughout the winter. During the warmer months, there are many more farmers' markets available and many farms also offer CSAs. CSA stands for Community Supported Agriculture. CSAs work like this. You pay ahead for the plan you want in mid to late winter. Many ask that you also donate a bit of your time to the farm over the course of the year and offer a variety of volunteer options to you. In return you get a weekly assortment of fresh produce throughout the harvest season. In most areas this will be from late spring through mid-fall. If you find a farmers' market or farm store in your area don't be afraid to talk to the farmers and ask about their growing practices and what kinds of fertilizers and pesticides they use, if any. Many small farms aren't certified organic because of the cost involved but are chemical free. Small farmers usually depend on their land for their livelihood and treat it with great care. Chances are, they are feeding their own family the same foods they are selling. Finally, if you live near the coast or large bodies of fresh water, you may also be able to get fresh, local fish and seafood. Again, ask about the fish you are buying. Is it wild caught or farmed? Is it local? Has it been frozen? It is your responsibility to make sure the food you buy for your family is of good quality.

When shopping for non-perishable items there are also options other than your local grocer where you can buy high quality, healthy food. One simple option is online stores. Many healthy, non-perishable food items can be purchased online for less than you would pay at your local market. Simply search "online food stores" and many options will come up. If you are comfortable with technology, you can easily search for items and compare cost and quality across several sites. Some offer free shipping with a membership or when your order reaches a certain dollar amount. Some membership-based companies offer trial periods for you to explore their website and make purchases before making a commitment. For non-perishable items, online shopping can be convenient and save you money.

With regard to food quality, in addition to freshness there are other things you may want to consider. Due to expanding agricultural practices in relation to the growing of food and feeding animals that are raised for human consumption, most whole foods and food ingredients fall into one of a few categories. In the produce department you may see produce listed as "conventional" or "organic". Conventional means that farmers are allowed to use chemical fertilizers, pesticides and weed killers, as well as genetically modified organisms (GMOs) for crop consistency. They also typically grow only one or two crops in each field, which depletes the soil of the nutrients used most by the crops grown. This poor soil results in produce that contains fewer nutrients than produce grown in soil that has not been depleted. Nutrient deficient produce provides less nutrition than more nutrient dense varieties produced by many small farmers and organic farmers.

Organic is defined as food grown on farms permitted to use only natural pesticides and natural fertilizers like manure. They also grow a variety of crops in the same soil or use cover crops in order to maintain high quality soil teeming with healthy nutrients. If a product is not identified as conventional or organic you can tell by the small sticker with the numbers attached to each piece of produce. These are price look up codes (PLUs) and are used internationally. Four-digit codes indicate conventionally grown items and five-digit codes identify organic items and have a 9 in front of the 4-digit conventional code for that item.

When purchasing non-produce items, you will often see Non-GMO, organic or both somewhere on the packaging. Non-GMO means the product is made from ingredients grown with no GMOs or very minimal amounts. The standards to be labeled Non-GMO are rigorous. Foods labeled Non-GMO are not organic, and may still contain ingredients grown with chemical fertilizers, pesticides and weed killers. All organic foods are also Non-GMO, but not all Non-GMO foods are organic. To be labeled organic, a product must contain at least 95 percent organic ingredients and any other ingredients must meet certain criteria to be used. If you don't see these labels, the product is most likely comprised of primarily conventional ingredients.

In general, the price of organic items is somewhat higher than their conventional counterparts, though this is not always the case. Some organic items are actually less expensive. Many grocery stores now carry a large variety of name brand organic items and many have their own generic organic options. You can often find a variety of organic and Non-GMO items listed in the weekly sale flyers. Read the fine print in the ads and look at the pictures. This is where you'll often see that an item is organic. Demand for organic food choices has increased dramatically and as a result many conventional farmers are converting to organic, which will increase the supply. As with other items, as the supply goes up, the cost will come down.

Depending on your family budget, you may be able to switch to an organic diet if you so choose. Most families who choose to purchase organic food items do not eat an entirely organic diet. If you'd like to start slowly or need to be choosy based on your budget consider the following information when planning which organic foods to purchase for your family.

There are many conventionally produced foods that are very safe and nutritious and our advanced sciences have been able to determine which foods tend to contain higher concentrations of harmful substances than others. These would be the conventional foods that you would want to replace with an organic variety. Meats and dairy products contain the highest amounts of residue because of their high fat content and the fact that they are high on the food chain. Pesticide residues tend to collect in fat and much of our livestock are fed diets consisting of high amounts of corn and soy, both GMO food crops in the United States. In addition, the majority of antibiotics used in the U.S. are used on animals. In reality, whatever the animal ate, you are also eating. Nuts and seeds, due their high fat content, also tend to be high in unhealthy substances like pesticides. It is healthiest to buy organic varieties when you can. Use this information to guide your food purchasing.

The next area to consider is fruits and vegetables. While not as high in residue levels as meats, dairy, nuts and seeds, most produce retains at least some of the chemicals used in the growing process. Thin skinned fruits and vegetables like grapes, apples and tomatoes contain more residue as a rule. Thicker skinned produce such as pineapples and melons, as well as foods like garlic and asparagus that attract few, if any, pests, contain lower amounts. Each year the Environmental Working Group, known as EWG, puts out a list of produce containing the highest and lowest amounts of harmful substances. It is updated annually and is available to the public on their website.

The final area to consider is grains. Even if not grown from GMO seed, almost all grains are sprayed with glyphosate, a synthetic herbicide, used at harvest to hasten the drying process in order to get them to market sooner. Most pastas, breads and cereals are made from grain products.

There is a lot to consider when making food choices for your family. Each family eats differently. If you are thinking of buying some organic foods, ask yourself what your family consumes in large amounts. That might be where you should start. If your children eat lots of fruit, start there. If they drink a lot of milk, start with milk. Start slowly. Over time you can increase the amount of organic food you buy. The overarching idea is to begin eating healthier.

Now that you know what to consider when buying food for your family, think about the organization of your local grocery store. When the focus is on serving real, whole foods to your family for meals and snacks, there are some shopping strategies that will help you. The majority of grocery stores are set up in a similar way. They typically have the real, whole foods you will be looking for primarily on the perimeter of the store, with processed and packaged foods in the center aisles. On the perimeter you will usually find the produce, meats, fish, dairy and cheese and fresh bread products. You will need to go into the center aisles for some products, such as nuts and nut butters, oils, vinegars and other condiments, canned fish, pasta and beans, crackers, and dry goods like flour and sugar and dried spices and herbs. You may also find you like to have some frozen vegetables on hand and will visit the frozen foods aisle for select items. You may find after adjusting to this new way of shopping that you spend less time in the store. You will be cutting out a lot of time in the center aisles, which tend to be more congested with other shoppers as many people purchase more processed food than fresh food.

After you've gotten used to this new way of shopping for food, I highly encourage you to include your children in selecting some of the foods you buy. I know it can be challenging taking children to the store with you and can seem like more work than it's worth, however, it has been found that children who help select the foods they eat, often eat a wider range of foods and are willing to try more things. Giving kids a voice in what the family will eat is a great way to give them some of the autonomy they seek. As an adult you are able to choose the activities you participate in, what you will wear and the food you will eat. Give your kids the same opportunity when it comes to some of their food choices. Strive to make this a positive experience for everyone. Plan your visit to the store with children shortly after a meal and when everyone is well rested, which will enable them to participate in a productive and enjoyable way.

The produce department is a great place to let kids help out. Giving younger children a choice between two or three things is a reasonable way to start. For example, let them choose what color apples you will buy that week. As kids get older, give them more choice and leeway. Challenge them to find different colored foods, so that they are eating a rainbow of color over the week or see if they can find a new fruit or vegetable that they haven't tried before. You be the guide and set the boundaries and let them make choices within your guidelines.

One final piece of advice is to avoid grocery shopping when you are hungry even if you are alone. People who shop when they are hungry tend to overbuy and buy things that they don't need. If you shop when you are hungry, even if you go with a list, you'll find that you leave with things you didn't intend to purchase. Shopping hungry can sabotage your healthy eating plan.

You're now armed with lots of knowledge and strategies to help you buy healthy, whole foods for your family. You know how to make a complete shopping list to avoid unnecessary trips to the store. You have a variety of places where you can purchase food, which include farmer's markets, CSA programs and online options. You know the importance of considering food quality when making decisions about what you're buying and you know that the majority of fresh, whole foods are found on the perimeter of the grocery store. It's now time to head out and get started!

Chapter Four

Putting It All Together

You've already done the planning, bought the food and started to stock your pantry. You're well on your way. The next step is making the meals you've planned. Stick to your menu and you'll be all set. Remember, you don't need to have a lot of cooking knowledge or a lot of kitchen supplies. You may have looked up some recipes during your planning or consulted a cookbook or two. You're set!

Go back to your menu. Are there some things such as casseroles, soups and other similar meals that you decided to prepare ahead of time, or want to make in big batches? If this is your plan, one strategy is to find a fairly large chunk of time, maybe on the weekend if your weekdays are busy with work and other activities. Estimate how long you think it will take you and then add some additional time. Most likely, if you are new to cooking from scratch, it will take you longer than you think at first. If you won't be eating the meals for several days, freeze them. You can freeze them cooked and plan to reheat them when you are ready to eat or freeze them prepared and cook or bake them just prior to serving. (If they contain meat or fish that was already frozen you must cook or bake the meal before refreezing.)

Many people take some time at the start of the week to

cut up fruits and vegetables so they are ready to eat. This encourages healthy snacking and makes grabbing a snack and packing lunches faster and easier. You'll want to purchase some stackable, reusable storage containers if you are going to do this. If you want your children to be able to have access to these, make sure the storage options you choose are manageable for them. It's useless to have healthy things cut up and ready for them, if they can't open the containers. Some families even go so far as to prepack sandwiches and other lunch and snack items and store them in labeled containers in the fridge. When it comes time to make lunches or snacks, it's easy to just grab what you need and package it up to go. School age children can even make their own lunches using this method. Label the storage containers using words or pictures, so kids know what's in each one. Make sure you've got one for each part of the lunch you want them to have and show them how to take one thing from each container, so they have a complete lunch. Having kids pack their own lunches provides a double bonus – they will be gaining independence and you will have more free time!

Just as including your kids in the process of selecting food at the store has its benefits, including them in food preparation and in making their lunches has benefits, also. When kids help prepare food, they are often more excited to eat it. If you can, include everyone in the food prep in some way. This doesn't have to be for every meal but letting them help even a few times a week is beneficial. It adds to the time your family spends together and builds children's language and social skills. It can be fun to have everyone preparing a meal together. Keep it simple. Tacos or pizza are both easy meals to let kids help prepare. If the whole family is a bit much in the kitchen, or you have small children, have one child help at a time. This gives you both some well-deserved one on one time. Involving kids in making meals and snacks is a fun way for them to add to their repertoire of skills. Even some of the simplest food preparations, such as making pudding, involve measurement. Preparing things that need to bake can improve their sense of passage of time. They'll also learn about healthy food choices and good nutrition in a natural and engaging way. Including kids in the kitchen is a great way for them to learn and practice important skills they'll use throughout their lives. By including kids in this way they'll discover that food preparation can be fun and you'll foster the importance of home cooking and eating real, whole foods. They won't be with you forever. Take the time to teach these skills and healthy habits now and there's a pretty good chance they'll take them with them when they go.

Children can help in the kitchen in many ways. The key is to match the job to the child. (See chart on page 28.) You know your children and their capabilities best, so use these suggestions as general guidelines. Kids who have never been in the kitchen before will need to start with simpler things even if they are older. For younger children and older children learning to cut, you can purchase training knives specially made for working on this skill in a safe way. They will still need adult supervision and some modeling, but it will get them started and foster feelings of accomplishment and independence. If you're new to the kitchen, too, learning these skills as a family will benefit everyone and take some of the pressure off you. Keep it low key and relaxed. Don't get fancy. Real, whole food ingredients and simple recipes make delicious meals and build healthy families.

Once you've started on this new venture and found some healthier dishes and snacks that your family really enjoys incorporate them into your meal plan regularly.

Suggested ways for kids to help in the kitchen:

Children aged 2 to 4	Children aged 5 to 8	Children aged 9 to 12	Children aged 13 and up
Put napkins, forks and spoons on the table Tear lettuce for salad Add nuts, seeds and precut ingredients to salad Add measured ingredients to recipes Stir pancake or cake batter, tuna fish and other salads Make trail mix Spread sauce and sprinkle ingredients on pizza Scrub vegetables	All of the things 2 to 4-year-olds can do plus: Set the table Make most of a salad Cut fruits and vegetables with a training knife Measure ingredients into cup measures Scoop/serve cold foods like yogurt, ice-cream, salads, cereals Help load and empty the dishwasher/help hand-wash dishes Get snacks and make cold sandwiches	All of the things 2 to 8-year-olds can do plus: Mix and make things like tuna salad, pancakes, brownies, cookies, oatmeal and grilled sandwiches Use the microwave Open cans with a hand or electric opener Load and unload the dishwasher except knives and other dangerous items Use the stove top with guidance Use regular knives with supervision	All of the previously mentioned plus: Cut and prepare fruits and vegetables Use the stove top independently Use the oven for baking Load and unload dishwasher Use a blender or food processor with guidance Pour and serve hot foods and beverages independently Make simple meals

Chapter Five

The Value of Dirt

You're probably wondering why the topic of dirt is in the food section of this book. Well, in order to build a truly healthy family you need to know some basics about the immune system and gut and, believe it not, dirt plays a significant role in building these two things!

First, a bit on the immune system. The immune system protects us from germs and chemicals that enter our body from the outside world. It also protects us from natural, cellular level changes that occur within our body. If left unchecked, these natural occurrences can turn into conditions like cancer. The immune system has two parts that act in conjunction with each other. One part is the innate immune system, which works at the cellular level mostly in the form of "killer cells" and "scavenger cells". These cells focus on bacterial infections and the naturally occurring cell changes that take place within all of our bodies that can put us in harm's way.

The second part is the adaptive immune system, which is really the body's learned immune system.

Depending on what antibodies have been delivered either through vaccines or exposure to certain illnesses, this immune system adapts and learns accordingly and is your line of defense against specific disease-causing organisms or viruses. This system is constantly learning and adapting giving it the ability to protect you against bacteria or viruses that change over time.

You should now have a greater appreciation for your immune system than you did just a minute or two ago. You can see how important it is to your overall health. Interestingly, the health of your immune system is, in part, dependent on the health of your gut.

Your gut is made up of bacteria known as the gut microbiome, which helps with digestion. Until recently, it was thought that digestive support was the only job of the bacteria in the gut. However, over the last several years it has become more and more apparent to scientists studying this area, that the immune system and the gut microbiome communicate, work together and have an effect on each other.

We now know that everyone has a unique microbiome. It begins before we are even born. Babies who are born vaginally, typically have stronger gut microbiomes than those born via cesarean section, because the birth canal is teeming with bacteria. Contact with these bacteria is important for the colonization of an infant's gut microbiome as is contact with other bacteria in the immediate surroundings directly following birth. Exposure to these bacteria during and directly after the birthing process increases the diversity and strength of the child's microbiome and immune system that they will carry with them throughout life. Breastfeeding helps to further colonize the infant's developing microbiome with flora from the mother. During the first one to three years of life, a child's gut is undergoing great change and development and will closely resemble that of an adult by age three.

The quality and diversity of the gut microbiome does not remain constant throughout life. It is adversely affected by a number of outside influences. One known fact is that the amount and variety of gut bacteria one has is related to diet. Gut bacteria seem particularly impacted by carbohydrates, or sugars, which feed fungi that promote such things as yeast infections and sinusitis. Eating simple carbohydrates like those found in products containing refined grains, like the white flour used in most baked goods, can adversely affect gut health, as can eating processed foods which contain high amounts of sugars and other ingredients that damage the microbiome. Meat products from poorly raised animals who are typically administered large amounts of antibiotics and fed GMO containing feed, also have a negative impact on gut health.

Another outside influence that affects gut bacteria is medication. It is now known that antibiotics not only kill the bacteria they are designed to attack, but the good bacteria in our bodies, as well. They are particularly damaging to our gut bacteria, which help support good immune function. In fact, just one week of broad spectrum antibiotics depletes the gut microbiome by approximately 25% and researchers have found that it can take as long as a year to rebuild it to its previous state. This is assuming no other bacteria depleting factors are introduced during the rebuilding period such as another round of antibiotics. During that rebuilding phase, while your gut is not equipped to work at full capacity, you are at risk of developing other problems. Additionally, it has been found that while the gut rebuilds itself over time, it may not regenerate completely and the outcome may yield a different, and possibly weaker, gut environment than what one had prior to the antibiotic treatment. Other medications can also cause changes in the gut microbiome, including NSAIDS (non-steroidal anti-inflammatory drugs), PPIs (proton pump inhibitors), laxatives and antidepressants. Not surprisingly, both smoking and alcohol consumption, also, adversely affect the gut microbiome causing disease to occur over time.

Another influence to be aware of is antibacterial products. Antibacterial products arose out of fear of bacteria and bacterial illness. People wanted to be more hygienic and decrease the risk of contracting bacteria related illnesses. Unfortunately, the ingredients that make anti-bacterial products effective against household bacteria and bacteria on the skin are detrimental to our gut bacteria, too. Anti-bacterial agents are found in such products as general household cleaners, including window cleaners and laundry soaps. They are found in hand sanitizers, soaps and hand lotions, toothpaste and mouthwash, plastic wrap, garbage bags and some household textile products including carpet underlay. You can't undo the past, but you can control the future. Be aware of what you are putting into your family's bodies, the personal care products you purchase and the products you are using in your home. Take this information and work toward maintaining your family's gut microbiomes. Carefully select the foods and products you purchase. Avoid those labeled antibacterial. Good hand washing with plain soap and water is the best way to safely rid ourselves of the dirt and bacteria we encounter on a daily basis and helps preserve our microbiome. Limit medications when you can and use antibiotics only when absolutely necessary. Stop smoking and stop or limit alcohol consumption. A diverse well populated, healthy gut is paramount to good health!

With just this basic knowledge about the human immune system and gut microbiome you can see how important both are to human health. The two are somewhat dependent upon one another and work together to maintain health. This is a very simplified explanation. The immune system is stimulated by an inflammatory response somewhere in the body. Many inflammatory responses begin in the gut, which is often referred to as the second brain. The two brains communicate and send messages back and forth to one another. Here is an example of how they communicate. The gut "brain" is triggered to message the brain in the head when inflammation sets in. The brain in your head, in turn, sends a message to the immune system letting it know there is some "invader" present. This signals the immune system to begin an attack on the "invader" in order to prevent or get rid of illness or disease that has set in. Understanding how the gut and immune system interact, allows you to see how when one or both are depleted, your health is affected. An unhealthy gut, doesn't have the strength and diversity needed to work properly and set this course of events in action. The end result can be illness, often chronic in nature, obesity or a host of other health problems.

Living a healthy lifestyle promotes a healthy gut microbiome. There are many simple things you can incorporate into your daily life to support this. One of the best things to do is eat a healthy diet comprised of real, whole foods. Be sure to include lots of vegetables, fruits, nuts and seeds, which provide lots of dietary fiber. Try to eat more vegetables than fruits because fruits contain natural sugars, which can be problematic if eaten in excess. When purchasing vegetables, consider how they were grown. Vegetables grown in good, healthy soil will contain lots of beneficial microorganisms. Refrain from scrubbing and peeling fresh vegetables. These two processes deplete the number of healthy microorganisms available to you when you consume them. If you are lucky enough to grow your own vegetables or buy directly from a farmer who uses responsible growing practices, just lightly rinse off any dirt, prepare and consume. The same goes with fresh, local fruit. Purchasing organic seeds and nuts is also a good idea if you can find them, as conventional varieties can retain high amounts of pesticides and other residue due to their high fat content.

If your family consumes meat, include responsibly raised meats in your diet. Grass fed, organic meats are the healthiest. Organic meat is from animals that were raised without the use of antibiotics and were fed non-

GMO feed. You'll also want to avoid conventionally produced corn and soy products and conventional canola oil. These are the largest GMO crops grown in the United States. Keep in mind that conventionally produced wheat products are sprayed with glyphosate at harvest to speed up the drying process and should also be avoided when possible. If sugar is an ingredient in products you buy make sure it is listed as pure cane sugar. Sugar beets are one of the newest GMO crops and are used in place of pure sugar to sweeten many foods. The same goes for sugar that you buy for baking and sweetening.

There are some foods that contain known probiotics. Probiotics are living microorganisms that have health benefits and directly impact the gut microbiome in a positive way. We all have large amounts of microorganisms living both in and on our bodies. Many foods contain natural probiotics that are similar or identical to the probiotic strains that inhabit the human body. Incorporating these foods into your diet is a surefire way to maintain a healthy microbiome. Probiotic containing foods are foods that are naturally fermented such as yogurt, kefir, sauerkraut, kimchi, pickles found in your grocer's refrigerator section, kombucha, raw cheese, apple cider vinegar, tempeh and miso. Tempeh and miso are both produced by fermenting soybeans and other ingredients. If you choose to incorporate these two foods into your diet, choose organic varieties. Incorporating lots of healthy, real food choices, including foods naturally high in probiotics will support your family's overall health.

If your family doesn't consume much in the way of

probiotic rich foods, supplements are available. Ideally, you want to get the nutrients you need from real food, however, you may want to add probiotic supplements to insure good gut health. It is also recommended that individuals on antibiotics include a probiotic supplement or plenty of probiotic rich foods in their routine while taking the antibiotic and for some time afterward in order to replenish the gut.

Probiotics have a close relative called prebiotics. Probiotics, being living microorganisms, need food like all other living things. Prebiotics, in addition to helping to prevent cancer and obesity, among other things, also feed probiotic microorganisms, thereby improving gut and immune system health. There are many foods that contain prebiotics. These include bananas, carrots, asparagus, yams, onions, garlic, tomatoes, radishes and leeks. Some other sources are flax and chia seeds, coconut meat and flour, chicory root and dandelion greens. Adding some of these prebiotic rich foods into your family's diet will further promote good gut health.

So where does dirt fit into all this? To appreciate the true health value of dirt we need to take a trip back in time. For thousands of years humans lived outside or in crude dwellings with earthen floors and walls and even roofs of soil. Living in this environment insured that they consumed a good deal of dirt. Today we don't live that way, but our bodies still benefit from contact with dirt either directly or by consuming food grown in healthy soil. Eating plenty of fruit and vegetables grown in healthy soil is good for you in many ways. The outside of responsibly grown produce is teeming with healthy bacteria. A light rinse is all that is needed before consuming. Avoid scrubbing and peeling. The soil of the past was of good quality. It hadn't yet been contaminated by man's attempt to keep bugs and weeds at bay. It was part of the human environment and played a significant role in maintaining human health. People didn't wash their hands several times a day. Dirt particles remained on their bodies and got in the food and water they drank. They consumed relatively large amounts of dirt and were all the healthier for it. Keep this in mind as you read the next few paragraphs.

A great way to keep your children healthy is to let them play outside regularly. Encourage outdoor play as often as possible. It can play a big role in maintaining the health of the microbiome. Provide opportunities for kids to roll in the grass, dig in the soil and jump barefoot in mud puddles. Letting them run barefoot in warmer weather is not only healthy for their foot development, but a great way to increase exposure to environmental microorganisms. The skin on the palms of the hands and the soles of the feet is highly absorbent compared to skin on other areas of the body. Refrain from using fertilizers and other chemicals in outdoor areas where your children may play, so that they can safely enjoy all of the benefits the natural environment has to offer.

Another noteworthy discovery is that it has been found that people who live with animals, dogs and cats in particular, tend to have more varied skin and gut microbiomes then those not living with animals. In a Canadian study, infants who were exposed to furry animals before birth and in early infancy had an increased diversity of healthy gut bacteria when compared to infants not living with animals. Children living with animals tend to develop fewer allergies and there is some evidence that gut organisms obtained through sharing a living space with animals decreases a child's chances of becoming obese as they get older. In addition to acquiring the microbiota carried by your animals, animals who go outside also bring microorganisms from the outside in. Playing with your dog or cat's feet after they've been outside, is another way to expose yourself to healthy organisms living outdoors. If you're an animal lover, a furry pet is a very healthy addition to your family!

Finally, children exposed to a wide variety of bacteria tend to be healthier overall. Allow young children to crawl and play on the floor. Don't panic if they put toys in their mouths. We all want to protect our children, but preventing them from contact with regularly occurring environmental bacteria is not helping them. Certain times of the year bring colds and other viruses. As much as you don't want to see your child under the weather with a cold, don't stay home because it's cold season. Protecting your young child from these viruses doesn't help them. Exposure to colds, viruses and germs through playing with other children in social settings, such as daycare centers and play groups helps them to develop stronger immunity. Children in daycare and those with siblings are naturally exposed to more germs and get more colds and viruses, which helps them build better immunity at a younger age than their counterparts who don't experience the same exposures. Children need to build up an immunity to the viruses that cause these ailments.

Catching a cold builds immunity to that particular virus and helps strengthen their overall immune system.

The take away – do all you can to help every member of your family build and maintain a healthy gut and immune system. They are instrumental to good overall health. You now know what types of foods deplete the gut microbiome and which ones help build and maintain it. Incorporate real, whole foods full of fiber and healthy microorganisms into your family's diet. Make sure to include prebiotic and probiotic rich foods on a regular basis. Add a furry friend or two to your family and don't worry about colds and other viruses. They help build healthy children. And, last, but certainly not least, always keep in mind that dirt is of great value when it comes to human health. From the prehistoric days to the present humans have lived with dirt. Expose your children and yourself to the outdoors and all the fun and dirt that come with it.

Chapter Six

The Importance of Movement

We all need to move every day. From the beginning of time humans were movers. For thousands of years, people moved throughout their day as they hunted and gathered food and searched for shelter and sources of water. The earliest people were hunters and gatherers and led a nomadic lifestyle, constantly moving from place to place in order to survive. They did little sitting. It wasn't until about 12,000 years ago, when the first grains were discovered growing in the middle east, that humans set up more permanent homes and became farmers. They did this because grains were the first food that they could store for periods of time and they could not store food if they were always on the move. Early farming was a lot of work and these early people continued to move the majority of the time.

Fast forward to the year 2000. The average person no longer has to hunt, gather or farm for their food. We simply go to a store, a restaurant or the nearest drive thru to get our next meal. Our jobs have many of us sitting at desks doing a variety of tasks for much of the day. While we are at work, our children are sitting in classrooms, often for stretches of a half hour or more without the chance to get up and move, with opportunities for movement decreasing with each consecutive year in school. Most people travel to and from work or school via modern transportation of one sort or another, which requires additional time spent seated. The majority of us then end our day sitting again. This time while we eat, socialize and relax in front of the television or computer to wind down in the evening. Our modern lifestyle requires very little movement, yet, movement is necessary for good health and survival.

Being physically active is one of the most important things you can do for your body. In order to be in good health, we all need to move. Physical activity affects all aspects of human health; body, mind and spirit. Movement helps keep these three facets of the human healthy and strong. The human body was meant to be active the majority of the time. The common saying, use it or lose it, puts the need for movement in perspective. We should use it as a motivator to be active even when we may not want to be. When we are young and healthy, we can choose whether to be active or not. However, as we age, if we don't stay active, our bones and muscles weaken and lose their strength from lack of use. Our stamina, or the ability to be active for more than a short period of time, diminishes. Chronic disease may set in. A time may come when we may no longer be able to choose whether to be active or not. Our body won't be able to be active because we did not keep it active over the years.

Many older people suffering from arthritis and other conditions that affect the body physically, pass them off as old age, however, if one stays active and works to keep their body strong and healthy, bones, joints and muscles stay strong. There are several zones in the world referred to as Blue Zones. The Blue Zones are areas of the world with the largest percentage of people not only living to see their hundredth birthday, but also living free of the chronic diseases that plague much of the modern, industrialized world. They don't suffer from obesity, type II diabetes, high blood pressure, high cholesterol, cardiovascular disease or cancer. One common characteristic of people living in Blue Zones is that they live very active lifestyles, often walking long distances daily, tending their gardens and participating in individual and group sports within their communities. Another common characteristic is that the elders remain active both within their families and in the larger community. In some of these areas there is no such thing as retirement. The word doesn't even exist in some languages. The lifestyle of these modern communities where people live long, healthy lives is evidence that remaining active is a necessity if you want to remain healthy.

Regular movement works to keep the human body healthy. Movement does a variety of things. As mentioned earlier, it helps to keep our muscles strong. Strong, healthy muscles allow us to be physically active in many ways without discomfort. This in turn builds endurance, or stamina, allowing us to be comfortably active for long periods of time. Think back to our ancestors, who traveled from place to place searching for food, water and safe shelter. They were active for many hours a day. In addition to helping maintain strong muscles, activities such as walking, running, jumping and climbing help build strong bones. These are known as weight bearing activities. When we do such things as walk, run and jump, new bone tissue is formed making our bones stronger. It is especially important for children through the teen years to be participating in all kinds of weight bearing activities because it is during childhood and puberty that the greatest amount of bone mass is gained.

Apart from muscle and bone strength, the body benefits from regular movement in several other ways.

Movement helps boost our energy levels during the day and supports good sleep at night. It helps maintain blood pressure and can even help decrease it. It increases your levels of HDL, known as the good cholesterol. It improves blood flow, so that all parts of your body get the oxygen they need to thrive. It helps us maintain a healthy weight and can support weight loss efforts in those who are overweight. Keeping these things in check reduces your risk of developing heart disease or suffering a stroke. Another benefit of regular movement, especially weight bearing activities, is the prevention of osteoporosis, a condition caused by loss of bone, which can result in fractures as we age.

Regular activity also supports the health of your mind and spirit. These two go hand in hand. When you are active, you are often happier. Have you ever wondered why? When we are active the feel-good hormones; serotonin, dopamine and endorphins, are produced and released. The feel-good hormones that are released are dependent upon the type of activity you engage in. All three promote positive feelings. This is why regular physical activity decreases stress, anxiety and depression. When you are feeling positive, you have a better attitude and outlook on life. Most people who are generally active feel good about themselves and their abilities, which enables them to weather life's up and downs with relative ease. Incorporating daily physical activity is critical in maintaining a healthy mind and spirit!

It's amazing how physical activity, or lack of it, can affect a human life. Think about an average day for most people. It probably doesn't include much physical activity. In general, we live a very sedentary lifestyle, especially when compared to the lifestyle of our ancient ancestors. In the introduction to this chapter, some of the aspects that limit our movement today were explored. Everything from the way we travel, to our jobs and the design of our educational system, to the way we obtain the things we need and the way we spend our "down time". Even the limited information presented in the first few pages of this chapter explaining how important movement is in order to maintain health, should make it apparent that today's lifestyle, with its limited opportunity for movement, is unhealthy. The rates of chronic disease are soaring in adults as well as in teens and young children. Many people are living with metabolic syndrome, characterized by a diagnosis of at least three of the following; being overweight or obese, especially around the mid-section, having high blood sugar, high blood pressure, high triglycerides and low HDL (the good cholesterol). Receiving a diagnosis of just one of these puts a person at higher risk for developing other health conditions including cancers.

I don't know anyone who wants to hear they have a chronic disease, yet many people aren't willing to become more active in order to maintain or improve their health. Most people have the attitude that it won't happen to them, until it does. The majority of people don't understand the real connection between activity level and disease. When asked, many people will say they know they should be more active, but also feel they deserve time to relax after working or going to school all day. They feel tired and worn out. They lack the energy and desire to be active. They feel overwhelmed by life's pressures and demands. They are stressed and anxious. Some are even depressed. Many people truly feel this way. What they don't realize is that they feel this way primarily because of the sedentary habits they have developed. It is because of the way they have spent their day and many days, weeks and months before this. They are living in bodies that are weak and depleted of energy. They lack stamina because they have been movement deficient for so long. Their lack of movement has inhibited the release of the feel-good hormones often resulting in a negative outlook and feelings of unhappiness and depression.

The good thing is, it's never too late to live a more active lifestyle. Replacing much of the time you and your family spend sitting while not at work or in school with some form of active movement can help reduce the risk of developing chronic health problems. If you or members of your family already have health issues, don't despair. Most physical and mental health problems, can be improved or even eliminated by consistently engaging in healthy amounts of movement daily.

Being physically active is as important to your health as the food you eat. Making sure you and your family are physically active every day is a major component to building and maintaining healthy bodies.

Chapter Seven

Movement and Exercise

Movement and exercise are similar but different. All exercise is movement, but not all movement is exercise. Movement could be defined as anything you do that is not sedentary in nature. Exercise is usually a planned activity resulting in higher amounts of energy expenditure.

Ideally, you want to add more general movement to your day. This can be quite challenging especially when you are first starting out. Many sedentary behaviors are habits and breaking habits is hard.

Take a few minutes to mentally go through your average day and then do the same for your family members. Do you spend a lot of time sitting or standing without really moving? You may not even be sure. If you and your family are like most average Americans, you spend much more time sedentary than actively moving about. Before trying to make changes, it's worth it to track sedentary time for an average day in your life. Most likely you'll be astonished! Here's one way to track a day. First, subtract the hours you usually spend sleeping from twenty-four. Then take the number of hours you are usually awake and multiply by sixty to get the total number of minutes you are up. To track an average day, record the number of minutes you are sitting or standing still. You can record them in your phone, on an index card or using some other small thing you can keep with you throughout the day. Make sure to record them in minutes. At the end of the day, tally up your sedentary time. Divide the total number of sedentary minutes by the total number of minutes you are awake on an average day. Move the decimal in your answer two places to the right and you've got your percentage of time spent sedentary.

Here's an example. If a person sleeps eight hours a night on average, they are awake sixteen hours each day. Multiply sixteen by sixty (minutes in an hour). That person is awake about nine hundred sixty minutes a day. They spent seven hundred forty-three minutes sitting or standing still. Divide seven hundred forty-three by nine hundred sixty and you get 0.7739. Move the decimal two places to the right and the number becomes 77.39. This person is sedentary seventy-seven percent of their waking hours.

Another way to assess your activity level is to track your steps. Most smart phones are equipped with a step counter and there are many apps that can be downloaded that include this feature. If you don't have a smart phone or other step tracking device, a simple pedometer can be purchased for less than ten dollars. You may want to purchase one anyway, as carrying your phone every step of the day, can be inconvenient. A pedometer is small and can be clipped to your clothing, so you don't have to worry about it.

If you choose to track your steps as a guide, the following information will help you judge where you currently fall with your movement. It is recommended that we take at least 10,000 steps a day for good health. This is equivalent to walking approximately five miles. This may seem outrageous to you, but remember how our ancient ancestors lived. They walked, ran, hunted and foraged much of every day just to survive. How many miles do you think they averaged a day? I'm thinking more than five!

Many groups have looked at daily steps taken by different groups of people and estimate that the average American takes between 4,500 and 6,000 steps a day, about half the recommended amount. Some even say these estimates are on the high side, indicating just how sedentary our modern lifestyle has made us. If you track steps, look at where you come out in relation to the average American and the recommended 10,000 steps per day. Your tracked steps are your baseline or starting point. Whether you choose to calculate sedentary minutes per day or track your steps, don't be discouraged if your sedentary percentage is high or your step count is low. You're not alone. As you build more movement into your lifestyle, track a day periodically to see your progress.

Children tend to be more active than adults by nature. Their short attention spans and generally high metabolisms have them moving quite a bit. They enjoy running and jumping. Even their quieter play often involves some movement. They will push toy cars along the floor, take their dolls or stuffed animals for a walk, or play dress up. These activities, while calmer in nature, all involve movement. Unless younger kids are involved in some sort of screen time activity, they tend to be at least somewhat active most of the time. Having young children walk around with a pedometer to track their activity level isn't necessary. You know what your child's typical day entails. You should be able to judge how sedentary they are. You can use the same formula provided earlier in the chapter for tracking their general sedentary time. Estimate the number of minutes they sit for their typical activities over the course of the day and plug in the numbers. If your children are older, you might buy them a pedometer if they are interested in tracking their steps. Creatively involving kids in activities, even those aimed at improving their health, makes them more inclined to try new things. Make it into a game or challenge, first establishing everyone's baseline and then working together to build more movement in for everyone.

Your goal should be to have everyone active the majority of the time. Aim for as little sedentary time as possible. The more active you are, the healthier you'll be. With a little effort, over time, you'll be moving more and sitting less.

Depending on your job, your commute and other aspects of your day, this may seem quite challenging. You likely can't change the way you get to work or the fact that there are some parts of your day that require you to sit, possibly even for long periods of time. There are probably many things you can change though.

What counts as movement? According to the World Health Organization (WHO), movement is any activity that exerts energy and is produced by the muscles. The WHO also states that inactivity is the fourth leading risk factor of global mortality and raises the risk of breast and colon cancers, diabetes and coronary artery disease considerably. Imagine if we all just moved a little more, how these risk factors would decrease!

Knowing that movement is any activity produced by the muscles resulting in use of energy, everything you do, other than sitting or standing still, counts! Most of the day to day activities of life require movement. It's a simple as walking to and from the car to go to work or run errands, carrying the laundry to the laundry room and loading the washer, helping the kids pick up their toys after dinner or straightening up the house. Think of the movement you engage in just by doing the mundane household tasks daily. People who hire others to do these and other jobs like yard maintenance, are really shorting themselves, unless they are replacing these activities with lots of physical movement. These daily responsibilities really support your health and keeping up with them will add to the time you spend moving.

If you have been living a sedentary lifestyle, start small. Every little bit counts. Each time you go to sit down, ask yourself if you really need to sit down. Is there something you could do right then to add a little more movement to your day? Another approach is to think about the things you do sitting most days. Are there some sedentary activities that you could limit or even eliminate by replacing them with something more active? We all like to relax, but that doesn't mean sitting on the couch watching television or sitting looking at social media for a couple of hours after dinner every night. What could you do to replace those sedentary activities? There are probably things around the house that could be done. Remember that being physically active will make you feel more energized and will improve your mood, so even if it's evening and you are feeling tired and cranky after a hard day's work, you'll benefit in several ways from choosing an activity that supports movement rather than sitting still. In the short run, you'll be improving your energy and mood and will be supporting better sleep that night, and in the long run, your choice of movement over inactivity will be helping you to stay healthy by decreasing your risk for chronic illness.

If you read this book in order, you've already read the food section at the beginning. If you incorporate regular food shopping and daily meal preparation into your lifestyle, you'll add more movement by just doing those things. Instead of sitting in the car to ride to a restaurant or pick up a pizza, you'll have walked through the grocery store or other market shopping for ingredients, lifted and carried bags, put ingredients away and will spend time putting those ingredients together to make healthy meals for your family. If you've taken the kids along to the store and included them in the meal preparation as was suggested, they've also increased their movement. The last three chapters of this book focus on time management as it relates to different aspects of health. If you choose to implement some of the suggestions with regard to time management, you'll likely find that, once again, you will be increasing the amount of time you and your family are moving.

Where does exercise fit into the picture? Exercise certainly counts toward your movement and has all the health benefits of movement in general attached to it, but don't think you have to start scheduling in work outs and join a gym. If that's your thing, go for it! But, if it's not, don't feel as if you have to suddenly become an exercise fanatic. By definition, exercise is usually referred to as a planned activity performed with the purpose of expending high levels of energy. Some people are naturally drawn to exercise and use it as a means to relieve stress, support weight loss goals and increase muscle tone and strength. Some people use exercise as a form of meditation and a time to think and others make it a social event, by joining a team or exercise group.

If you're looking to increase your movement and enjoy particular sports or forms of exercise it's a great way to achieve your goal. However, exercising for a half hour or an hour doesn't take the place of regular movement throughout the course of the day. Studies have found that those who actively exercise, but then engage in sedentary behaviors the rest of the day, don't decrease their risk of chronic disease. Chronic disease risk reduction is attained through regular movement throughout the day, which certainly can include more formal exercise.

Being physically active throughout the day is a necessary component to staying healthy and reducing one's risk for chronic disease. It's as important for a two-year-old as it is for an eighty-two-year-old. It's also just as important as eating well. Real whole foods and consistent movement throughout the day are key factors in maintaining health at every age.

Chapter Eight

Building a Life of Movement

Now that you know how important movement is to your family's health, how do you make sure everyone is moving more? If your family is like the average American family, more movement is a must. Sedentary habits need to be broken and replaced with new habits that involve more activity. This will take some time as habits are hard to break.

If you haven't assessed where you and your family are with regard to movement, start with that. Think about what your family engages in that keeps them sedentary. It may be different for different family members. Do some quiet observing. You could do this over a week or so. Make sure to include estimated sedentary time at school or other places. If you've got little ones, they are probably pretty active during many of their waking hours whether they are in a day care setting or at home. It is likely that school-age children are sitting more throughout the day than is healthy. Elementary students have a lot of movement breaks built into their day as their short attention spans require teachers to change the activity regularly. Transitioning from one activity to another often requires that children get up and move to another place in the room. Elementary teachers also try to give children opportunities to be on the floor, at tables or up and moving around. As children begin middle school and move from class to class throughout the day, instruction becomes less movement oriented and students tend to sit for longer periods of time. Many may be sitting for as long as forty to forty-five minutes at a stretch. Opportunities for regular movement may be limited to the time they have between classes. This trend continues into the high school setting and unfortunately has our eleven to eighteen-year-olds, spending much of their day sitting still. If you and other adults in the family work at a career, you are probably also spending much of your day inactive. This lack of movement is part of the society we live in and is a direct result of the way our educational system and the majority of work systems are set up. The sedentary time spent at school and work are probably not easily modifiable by you, so we'll call it non-negotiable.

When evaluating your family's sedentary habits remember to consider what family members do after work and school. Does anyone participate in other activities out of the home? Do you stop to shop or run errands? Do your children participate in after school programs or sports? The types of activities everyone is involved in will affect the amount of time spent sedentary.

As you observe and think, make a list so you have something to go by and refer to. Writing something down also makes it more concrete, or real. Once you have your list, it's time to decide what to tackle first. Such things as the age of your children, your family's schedule, the amount of unscheduled, negotiable time available, the jobs held by the adults in the household and other factors, will, in part, govern the amount of sedentary time members are spending and will affect how you proceed.

Increasing the movement of younger children will probably be easier than that of older ones. Young children often adapt to change more easily. They are not as set in their ways and you have more control over what they do and how long they spend on activities. In most families, one of the biggest robbers of movement is the screen. It doesn't matter what type of screen; television, computer or phone. Technology has us sitting spellbound for hours staring at screens. Screen time will be covered more later in the book, however, it may be one of the key factors that is limiting your family's movement. Even the youngest of children are experiencing extensive amounts of screen time. There is programming for every age available at any time of the day or night. If screen time is one of the big culprits in your family, you need to start thinking of ways to limit it. When people aren't sitting in front of a screen they are generally more active.

Regardless of the type of movement robbers affecting your family and the extent to which movement is already occurring, there are very few people who don't need to move more. Movement is a necessity for good health. Time needs to be built into everyone's schedule for activities that involve movement. Everyone needs to spend time engaged in things that have them up and moving daily. Time spent moving decreases and counteracts time spent inactive.

Once again, start small. You've identified the things that are keeping your family members from moving more. Choose one thing to change, limit or add. Be specific. When we are specific, we are more likely to be successful. Actually write it down and post it somewhere if you think that will be helpful and more motivating. Building more movement into your family's lifestyle may be different for each person. It may be easier to start with one thing for the kids and another for yourself. Depending on what you choose, it may lend itself nicely to extra movement for everyone. You might decide that after dinner each night the whole family will help clean up and then find two things around the house that need to be put away. Right there you've probably added about ten to fifteen minutes of time spent moving. Maybe you decide to fit in a short family walk each day before or after dinner. Everyone participates. Maybe the kids ride their bikes or scooters while the adults walk. Adding in an activity like this could add a half hour or more of movement to everyone's day. Another way to get everyone moving could be to assign "jobs" connected to getting dinner ready. The adults may do the food prep, but kids can set the table, help make a salad and feed the cat or dog. Once again, everyone is up and moving.

Being outside often increases overall activity levels. When kids are home after school or on the weekend, outside play should be encouraged. When children are outdoors they are usually quite busy. If they sit, it will likely not be for long. Something will grab their attention and have them running to check it out. Invest in some outdoor toys and equipment for them. There are lots of inexpensive things for kids to use outside that also encourage active play such as jump ropes, bubbles, chalk, balls and hula hoops. Visit your local department store, sporting goods store, or go online for more inexpensive outside play ideas. Include your children in selecting new toys or activities for when they are outside. Again, giving children some say in what they do, in this case, how they spend their outdoor time, will have them excited and more likely to respond positively. Many children enjoy being able to move about on wheels and enjoy scooters, tricycles, bicycles, and other ride on toys. You may also consider purchasing larger items such as a basketball hoop, goals for soccer and hockey or a swing set. What you purchase, will all depend on your children and their ages.

Many items intended for outdoor use by children are very sturdy and will still be in good shape after children outgrow them. It may be worth your time to explore yard sales and thrift shops to see what you can buy used. If your children aren't used to outdoor play and you aren't sure what will interest them this may be the best way to start. Some kids latch on to one thing and never tire of it, while others need a variety of options and bounce from one activity to the next. Some children are very creative and can entertain themselves, while others need actual things for entertainment. Having a variety of activities for them to do outside is the key and will keep them moving.

As far as indoor ideas, things such as playing a board game together at the table, will have kids more active and engaged. Even if they're sitting they will be moving around a bit as they take their turn. If you've got a deck or two of cards around, teach them how to build houses from cards on the floor. They'll be on their knees and moving up and down as they try to find the best way to place the cards. If you have young children, there are many toys that can be used indoors that encourage pushing, pulling, climbing or balancing. When you are purchasing toys, keep these things in mind. Another idea, is to keep old blankets around for kids to make into forts, tents and other "places" to set up and play in. This type of activity will often keep children entertained for quite some time. You may have a large basement area available for more active indoor play where they could use balls, jump ropes and other outdoor toys inside. Be prepared for life to get a little crazy and loud. It does when kids are happy and playing. Remind yourself that active kids are healthy kids and just enjoy the busy hum of your active household.

Children old enough to play sports, may enjoy being part of a team. Explore what is available through your child's school, your local recreation department or other programs in your area. Dance, gymnastics and swimming are also great activities for kids. These tend to be more individualized, which some children prefer. Being part of a children's theater group may be another possibility. Find out what is available in your area for school aged children. Encourage your child to choose one extracurricular activity. Be careful not to overschedule children. They need a balance of structured and unstructured opportunities. If your child is older, two structured activities per week may be manageable. They might choose one sport related activity and another like scouting or an art. If your child chooses a team sport, that may be the only thing they should do. Find out how many practice sessions and games are scheduled each week. Getting involved in too many things causes stress and anxiety. You can end up with overlap of activities, especially on weekends and find your family running from one thing to the next with no time to breathe in between. One or two organized activities at most, are beneficial in many ways, and will keep your children moving in one way or another while insuring some unstructured play time as well.

Another way to get kids more active is to give them a few age appropriate chores to do. Even the youngest of children can help pick up toys, fold towels, match socks and carry small things to their room. Older kids can be required to make their bed, pick up their clothes and toys, bring clothes to the washer, help fold and put clean clothes away, dust, help load or empty the dishwasher, or wash dishes. They can help make lunches and get backpacks, shoes and coats ready for the morning. If your family has outdoor space to maintain, children can help outside, also. They can sweep, rake, shovel, water plants and more. The goal is to give them things to do that keep them up and moving.

When your family is out and about, use such strategies as parking toward the back of the lot at the store rather than the front to encourage more walking. If you have several errands in one area, park the car and walk from place to place. Use stairs and not elevators. Better yet, if you live within walking distance of where you need to go, walk or bicycle there.

Planning family activities is another way to build more movement into your family's lifestyle. Make them fun and exciting. Perhaps you build a treat in along the way or at the end.   One idea is biking. Many areas have beautiful bike paths to provide safe areas for biking, skating and walking. There are many seating options to include even the youngest members of your family in this activity. You might also find interesting areas to walk or hike. There are probably many options not far from home. Other fun activities to try are bowling or roller skating. If you live near the coast or a large body of water, go to the beach. Digging in the sand, building castles, swimming and playing in the water are all great ways to move. Beaches usually offer ample room for running and exploring. Beaches, bike paths, and other walking or hiking areas are fun year-round and offer different experiences by season. If you live in an area with a cold winter season try ice skating, sledding or tubing together. Another option, is to purchase a family membership to a local recreation center. Recreation centers offer numerous activities and opportunities and may be a good choice if you have older children who are beyond playing with toys. There are exercise classes and equipment they may be interested in trying. Many offer indoor pools and gyms. They may have open rec times when older kids can join in a basketball or floor hockey game. They usually offer something for everyone, including childcare and children's activities, so that everyone can participate in something they enjoy.

There are so many ways to build more movement into your family's lifestyle. They key is to start with something small and easily attainable. If you children, you may share with them that as a family you need to become more active and include them in the planning. The may have some great ideas. You may also choose to be creative and little by little build more movement in, without them really knowing that you're doing it. Be prepared to face some resistance at first with whichever method you choose. Breaking habits takes time. If your children are used to watching television right after dinner, they may balk when you change the routine. If they aren't used to playing outside, it will take some time for them to adjust to this new aspect of their life.

With consistency and perseverance these new habits will become part of your daily routine. Plan to work at each new strategy every day for several weeks. Consistency pays off. If your movement strategy involves an outdoor activity, decide that it will happen on rainy days. Will you all head outside anyway, or have an alternate plan for days when the weather doesn't cooperate. Establishing new habits or routines generally take a dedicated person at least three weeks. You are trying to make changes within your family, so expect it to take even longer. Write down your goal and be consistent and persistent. It will happen. Once you reach your goal and the movement has become routine, it's time to reward everyone and set your next movement goal. Before long, you'll be amazed at how much more active you all are! Every little bit counts. Try to keep everyone active the majority of the time you have at home and you'll all be on the road to better health!

Chapter Nine

Overscheduled Kids and Parents

Life in the present day can overtake you. It just happens to many of us. There are so many things we "need" to do each and every day. The majority of adults work out of the home, and most kids are educated in schools. On top of work and school, there are a myriad of other responsibilities and opportunities vying for our time. There are errands to run, bills to pay, meetings, practices and games to attend, homework to be done, meals to be eaten, lunches to be made and social engagements to be attended. I could go on and on. Every family is different, but most families are leading a rushed and stressful life much of the time and every member is affected. In order to have the healthy family we are striving for, we need to learn to manage time better.

Part of time management is being mindful. Mindfulness, in its true sense, refers to being present in the current moment and not thinking about the past or the future. Families need to apply the concept of mindfulness when deciding how to schedule their time. They need to be mindful first and foremost of everyone's health. Good health is the result of a high-quality diet, daily movement, adequate sleep, a relaxed body and mind and solid social connections. When planning how time will be spent, care must be taken to make sure each of these components can be met. These are imperative if we are to maintain the physical, emotional and spiritual health of each and every family member.

Think about your family for a minute. If your family is like most families today, you are probably overscheduled. You might not even realize it. You've been going along at a busy pace for months or even years. It's time to take a step back and look carefully at your family's schedule. The best way to do this is to track an average week or even a month in your family's life. You'll want to include work and school/daycare schedules, extracurricular activities for both the adults and kids in your home. These may include religious, exercise and other types of classes, scouts, sports, meetings such as PTO/PTA and school events. Jot down everything that is scheduled and takes time. If you recorded and analyzed sedentary time for your family you may be able to use that information. You'll also want to include which family members are involved in what activities, how many days each week the activity occurs, how long the activity is and the hours of the day it takes place. It might be a good idea to assign each person in your family a color and track their activities using their color. Using different colors will make it easy to see how busy each person is at a glance. Record time spent at work and school/daycare in a separate color. These are your non-negotiables. It might be good to record these in black. Once you've recorded your family's schedule tally up the time each person is involved in activities other than work and school/daycare over the course of a week. Then ask yourself these questions; How many activities do they have in a week? What types of things are they doing? Are they all similar or are they varied? Are they activities they chose to do? Are they enjoying them?

Now estimate how many waking hours each family member is not at work or school/daycare. Subtract the hours they spend participating in various activities.

Next, estimate the time it takes to prepare for the activity (get dressed, gather materials and equipment etc.). Include travel time to and from. Now subtract that. What's left is the amount of time each person has available for eating, homework, household responsibilities and chores, free choice activities and down time. You may be surprised now that you've got it all written down. It may have just become clear why you are all feeling so overwhelmed and exhausted. This awareness will help you in restructuring your family's lifestyle.

While it's important to expose children (and adults) to new experiences, to be active, and to participate in enjoyable activities, being overscheduled can have dire consequences. Many adults and children are on the run constantly. Their packed schedules don't allow them to be able to cook or eat a meal in a relaxed way. They may be lacking the time to get sufficient and varied movement into their day. They may not have time to socialize with friends or family members. In some cases, the overscheduling is a result of unspoken competition, or feeling obligated to join particular groups or activities. Many people feel they need to keep up with everyone else. They want to be accepted into, or remain part of, certain circles. At the end of the day, people are left feeling exhausted and sometimes unfulfilled. They have no time to relax and rejuvenate. Couples don't have time to connect. Parents and children don't have time to connect. There is little or no rhythm and routine within the family. Over time this negatively impacts the health and wellness of everyone.

What are the negative impacts of overscheduling?

Being overscheduled can cause stress and anxiety for adults and children alike. It can also be the cause of poor eating and sleep habits. Each of these alone can affect our health, but together they can significantly affect overall health and functioning.

Everyone has dealt with some stress and anxiety along the way, and in all honesty, a little bit here and there is good for us. It can help us learn how to deal with difficult situations and reassure us that we are capable of managing and overcoming stressful times in our lives. In days gone by, childhood wasn't depicted as a stressful time, yet spend some time with a group of children today and you will hear that they have a lot of worries. They worry about finding time for homework. They worry about practices and games. Much of their worry is due to the busy schedules they have. They are stressed. More and more children and teens are being diagnosed with stress and anxiety disorders. Even our youngest family members can be plagued by this.

Busy schedules often result in poor eating habits. Ideally, we should eat a good deal of time before we head to bed and our meals should be comprised of healthy, real, whole foods enjoyed in the company of others. Overscheduled families often have no set time for meals. Meals are often eaten on the go. On the go food is typically not very healthy. Too often it is takeout from a fast food restaurant or prepackaged, processed food that can be prepared quickly. Families are eating in the car, on bleachers, or very late in the evening. There's a good chance that when families do eat at home, televisions, video games and phones are the mealtime entertainment, rather than conversation with other family members. Once established, poor eating habits are difficult to change and over time will most likely lead to a lifetime of poor health plagued by chronic disease.

An extremely busy lifestyle also often results in poor sleep habits for adults and children alike. Many adults get up in the morning unrefreshed, wondering how they will get through another day. They spend their days feeling overwhelmed by the number of things they need to accomplish. Their schedules keep them in overdrive. Thoughts run through their heads from the minute they wake up to the minute they go to sleep. Unfortunately, many lay in bed night after night waiting for sleep to come, knowing that in just a few short hours the craziness will begin all over again. Their minds aren't able to slow down and relax enough for them to get the seven to eight hours of sleep that their body requires. It is during sleep that the body rejuvenates, repairs and cleanses itself of unhealthy toxins. Adequate sleep is imperative in maintaining good health.

It isn't just moms and dads who have poor sleep habits. Late meals and hectic schedules that run into the evening lead to kids getting to bed later than they should. Many kids are also running in overdrive as a result of their busy days, which has the same impact on their sleep as it does on the sleep of adults. They are expected to come home from an activity where they were probably quite active in a brightly lit area and get ready for bed. Lack of time to relax and slow down before going to bed often results in children lying awake long after the lights are out. As with adults, children's bodies are not given the time they need to rest and repair, so that they can wake up refreshed and ready to face the new day. Instead, they are tired and sluggish, making it difficult for them to eat, dress and get out the door on time. A tired body and brain have trouble focusing and learning. Kids caught in this cycle often have trouble in school, trouble with friends and difficulty managing their emotions. If this lifestyle persists their health eventually suffers.

Establishing an evening bedtime routine is key in helping everyone get the sleep they require. It should be predictable and include downtime and quiet, relaxing activities away from screens. Avoid keeping bright lights on, as this signals the brain to be active rather than to slow down. Use table lamps and bulbs with lower wattages and more filtered light in the evening. A warm bath or shower followed by a bedtime story or reading sets the body up for the healthy sleep necessary to be ready for the next day's adventures.

As adults, we are responsible for managing, to the best of our ability, the health and wellness of ourselves and our children. Less is often more when it comes to our family's schedule and how we manage negotiable time. Less structured time away from home leaves more unstructured time at home. It leaves time for connecting as a family, sharing meals together and hearing about each other's day. It leaves time to relax and enjoy some quiet time before heading to bed. We all thrive on structure and a predictable, unhurried evening routine will have everyone to ready for sleep and to bed at a reasonable time.

Managing a family's schedule is not a simple job. It can easily get out of control, often without anyone even realizing it until you find yourself and your family crazed by the life you are leading; a life that's too busy, a life that lacks daily routine and predictability, a life that makes connecting with others challenging, a life of meals on the run punctuated by fractured sleep. Putting the brakes on and taking the time to figure out what activities are truly worthwhile for your family will make life easier and more enjoyable. Less stress, healthier meals and rejuvenating sleep will do everyone a world of good!

Chapter Ten

Finding A Balance

Life is a balancing act. It always has been and always will be. A truly balanced life needs just the right amount of this and just the right amount of that. When life is well balanced, we experience happiness and peace. We are relaxed and fun loving. We have energy to do the things we want to do. We are able to make good choices, persevere and are resilient when faced with difficulties. We experience the gift of good health. It is life as it was intended to be.

What's difficult is finding and maintaining this delicate balance, while managing the day to day experiences that life throws at us. However, in order to insure the health of the body, mind and spirit needed to live life to its fullest, it's imperative that we find this balance both for ourselves and our children.

Modern conveniences such as electricity, automobiles, televisions, computers and microwaves have made life easier for us, but they have also greatly contributed to the demise of our health. Electricity has made it so that we have light whenever we want it. We no longer sleep based on earth's natural ebb and flow of light and darkness. Many household duties that used to require physical effort and movement are now accomplished by turning on an electric appliance of some sort, diminishing the amount of movement opportunities we naturally encounter in a day. Automobiles have made travel easy and fast. We no longer have to walk or use slower modes of transportation like horses and buggies, to get from place to place. We can go further, faster, which puts so many more opportunities within easy reach. However, this busyness can create stress. Automobiles and other modern-day transportation also contribute to our sedentary lifestyle and decrease the time we spend active. Televisions provide entertainment and news instantly, so we no longer need to socialize with others for entertainment and to learn of current events. Computers have put the world at out fingertips. The click of a mouse brings us whatever information we are seeking and even enables us to purchase items right from the comfort of our own homes. This same technology has made it possible to "go to work" without ever leaving home. The convenience the computer has afforded us, impacts our health further by, again, limiting the necessity for movement and general socialization with others. It minimizes the need to put much mental effort into thinking or solving problems. With just about every answer a click away we don't have to wonder about anything for more than a few seconds. It's all readily available on the nearest electronic device. Last, but certainly not least, microwaves have made the preparation of meals fast and easy. You can simply open a box, quickly heat the food and have a hot meal ready in no more than a few minutes. What's lost here in terms of health? Movement, nutrient rich meals from real, whole foods, and the opportunity to make meal prep a time to socialize with friends and family or a time to slow down and just get lost in our own thoughts. Many of the chronic health issues people are trying to manage have been brought about because we live in this modern era.

How do we find a balance? In creating balance be mindful of the elements a body needs to be healthy; good nutrition, regular sleep and movement, quality social connections and time to relax and reboot on a regular basis. When making decisions for your family ask yourself, "Will this contribute to, or take away from, my family's health?" Life choices that require us to be too busy, feel stressed, have poor eating and sleep habits and not get enough movement take away from our family's health. Over time, these all lead to systemic inflammation, which in turn leads to chronic disease. People have come to expect certain conditions such as type II diabetes, high blood pressure, high cholesterol, weight gain and cardiovascular disease to arise as part of the aging process. These chronic diseases are brought on, primarily, by living an unhealthy lifestyle. Conversely, they are all preventable when we consistently make good lifestyle choices. An unfortunate reality is that these diseases are no longer diseases of adulthood. More and more young people are being diagnosed with these very conditions and it's all because of the lifestyle we have created; one of convenience and ease. If members of your family are already dealing with one or more of these conditions, there is an upside. They can be improved and sometimes even eliminated from a person's life by adopting a balanced lifestyle. Keep in mind, those living in the Blue Zones rarely experience chronic disease. Follow their example. By consistently providing the body with the nourishment it needs through adequate food, movement, sleep, social connections and relaxation it becomes balanced. When the focus becomes finding and maintaining a healthy balance in the way you experience life, inflammation decreases. Most, if not all, chronic disease is a result of systemic inflammation. A decrease in inflammation, in turn, supports the body's effort to restore health. As health is restored, symptoms of chronic disease diminish. This all happens when we make mindful choices for ourselves and our children with regard to most everything we do. Even if your family is free of diagnosed chronic disease, it is very unlikely that systemic inflammation is not present to some degree. If a body is living in the fast lane, consuming any processed foods at all, not getting regular movement throughout the day (think 10,000 steps!) or not getting at least seven hours of sleep every night, systemic inflammation is present. As a parent, you shape your child's lifestyle with the choices you make for him or her every day, starting at birth. Making mindful choices for your children regarding food, sleep, movement and social interactions will set them on the right course for their future and the development of chronic disease will be unlikely. With that in mind, it's time to start finding that delicate balance for you and your family.

Busy families need a schedule. A well-planned schedule promotes health in every way for everyone. It takes into consideration the sleep and nutrition requirements of all members and insures that everyone is active throughout the day. It, not only, includes time for connecting with each other and fostering a healthy social network of friends and extended family, but also time for both the body and the mind to relax. A well-built schedule is predictable, provides structure to our days, keeps us rooted and helps insure that our family is getting what it needs in terms of a healthy lifestyle.

When planning for your family there are a few key ideas to keep in mind. In no particular order, they are; less is often more, well balanced schedules help keep us healthy, everyone benefits from a balance of structured and unstructured time, free play is valuable and screen time and social media are negatively impacting overall health.

While we all want the best for our children, we need to keep in mind that less is often more. When we have fewer responsibilities outside of work and school, we can devote more time to what really matters. A less busy schedule allows for more homecooked meals, more time for unstructured free play, which supports the imagination and creativity so abundant in children and a less stressed lifestyle. It allows for more opportunities to move about actively and freely, to connect with family, friends and neighbors and to relax as needed throughout the day. Consistent mealtimes and bedtimes with predictable routines not only promote physical health, but also result in a more relaxed atmosphere, which promotes mental and spiritual health for parents and kids alike. Fewer outside obligations allow us more time to get the necessary things accomplished in an unhurried way and still have time left in the day to devote to our own needs or interests. When life slows down, you will find that happiness, energy and resilience result for everyone.

We all need structure. It provides the organization and predictability we need to live in peace. When there is no structure, chaos and stress result. A schedule provides structure, but within the schedule it is important to make sure there is a balance between structured and unstructured time for all. Think of structured time as time spent engaged in particular, planned activities. It could be soccer practice, it could be homework, it could be doing chores, or even attending a meeting or class. Unstructured time is time that allows us to choose what we will do. We all need our days to include both structured and unstructured time.

For many children, the majority of their playtime is structured. Structured play involves participating in an activity orchestrated by a coach, leader or some other authority figure. It has established rules, routines and expectations. Children are expected to stay within the parameters set by "rules" of the activity. There is little or no room for creativity or thinking outside the box. For example, if they are on a soccer team, they are following the directions of a coach, playing by the rules of the game and are expected to be participating in the singular activity of soccer in the area assigned. If their attention is suddenly grabbed by a tree on the sidelines, they can't freely run off the soccer field to go explore the tree. Perhaps they could do so after the practice or game, but when the moment of wonder appears, they are "locked" into the structured activity of soccer. There are certainly benefits to participating in structured activities such as learning good sportsmanship, learning to play by established rules, learning to take direction and learning patience and turn taking. While some structured play is good, our minds and spirits are nourished through the types of opportunities that present during free play opportunities.

For children their unstructured hours should be a time for free play. In November of 1989, the United Nations Convention on the Rights of the Child was adopted by the UN General Assembly. Countries belonging to the United Nations agreed to recognize that all children have a right to play. Play England, a registered charity in England devoted to insuring that all children have the right to play throughout childhood, which encompasses the teenage years, defined free play as, "… children choosing what they want to do, how they want to do it and when to stop and try something else. Free play has no external goals set by adults and has no adult imposed curriculum. Although adults usually provide the space and resources for free play and might be involved, the child takes the lead and the adults respond to cues from the child."

Free play is probably one of most important things you can provide your child. Creating a schedule that allows for plenty of free play, is crucial to the social and brain development of children. Free play may or may not involve toys or other tangible things. It is during this unstructured time that children can unleash their creativity and imagination. It's during free play that the building blocks or crayons and paper come out. It's when kids have time to build forts and sandcastles. Clouds become dinosaurs, toads and fireflies are captured and hide and seek is played. Rocks are thrown into water to see how high the splash will be and over time kids will take on the challenge of learning to skip those stones along the water's surface and invite others to play along in a friendly competition. Imagine a childhood without time for these and other activities that stimulate the growing brain and contribute to lifelong learning!

Free play promotes problem solving. When other children are involved, it cultivates language skills, working with others, learning about perspective and becoming a flexible thinker. Free play is usually relaxed play and allows children the needed break from the parts of life that have parameters and expectations attached; the parts of life that can be stress promoting. However, free play also offers children opportunities to take risks, which in turn help them to develop confidence. A well-designed family schedule provides a healthy balance of structured and unstructured time with plenty of opportunities for free play.

When planning for your family, make sure to include some unstructured time for grownups, too! Having the opportunity to engage in activities with others that bring joy and relaxation are just as important for adults. Take time to interact in a playful and enjoyable way with your children, pets and significant other. When did you last sit and color with your child?

When did you last take your teenager for an ice-cream?
When did you last sit with your spouse and reminisce or
talk about your dreams for the future? Take time to be
with yourself, too. Enjoy some time reading, crafting
or just plain relaxing with a cup of tea. Allow your
brain some time to be creative and dream. When you
regularly include personal downtime in your schedule
and make time to do the things you love and the things
that you find energizing and fulfilling, you'll be happier
overall and better able to fulfill life's responsibilities.

So, where do you start? The area that probably
needs the most significant attention and managing is
your family's screen time. Screens have become an
integral part of our lives. They are everywhere. They
are all over our homes. They are part of our work,
school and play environments. They are even in our
cars! For many of us they are our window to the world.
They bring us the news. They bring us the faces of
family members living in distant places. We can
communicate with others both near and far almost
instantaneously. Screens are often the first thing we
look at in the morning and the last thing many of us
check at night. However, they are impacting our health
in a variety of ways.

Take a minute to think about all the factors that
you know are important for good health; good nutrition,
quality sleep, regular and varied movement throughout
the day, solid social connections and time for the body
and mind to relax and rejuvenate. Screen time can
negatively impact every one of these areas causing
many of us, young and old alike, to unknowingly
sacrifice good health.

For some reason, most of us become glued to screens easily. What was intended to be a quick check of our email or a text turns into extensive amounts of time spent scrolling and clicking. Even young toddlers know how to scroll through mom or dad's photos or find a "game" they like to play on the phone. Today's children are very adept with technology. They, like adults, get wrapped up in it very quickly and easily and one show or game turns into two or three and before long their entire afternoon or evening has disappeared while they were staring at a screen.

This doesn't seem so bad. It's a way to spend time, communicate and learn. Screens are part of our modern lifestyle and they are here to stay, but we need to find a healthy balance between screen time and other activities in order to maintain the delicate balance of health in a world where it is very easy to become unhealthy. Once again, it all comes down to making the right choices.

Before we can make choices about things, we need to know what to consider. I hinted earlier that screen time is not beneficial to our health. It's unhealthy in several ways. When we have our eyes fixed on a screen, there's a pretty good chance we are sedentary. If you're going to get those 10,000 or more steps in daily, you can't spend a lot of time engaged in behaviors that impede movement. Screen time is one of the biggest, if not the biggest, inhibitor of regular movement for kids and adults. Take the screens away from people and chances are they'll be moving about. The only time of the day we should not be engaging in regular movement is when we are asleep. Interestingly, many people also experience sleep difficulties. One culprit, you guessed it, is screen time. Screen time can affect sleep in different ways. First, the blue light emitted from most electronic devices can impact one's ability to go to sleep. Blue light interferes with the production of melatonin, the sleep hormone. When you are exposed to blue light too late in the day and melatonin production is limited, sleeplessness occurs. Significant exposure can even alter one's circadian rhythm, our natural sleep and wake cycle which is regulated by earth's natural cycle of light and darkness. If the circadian rhythm becomes unregulated significant health problems can result.

Screen time can also cause our bodies to be in the fight or flight mode rather than the rest and restore mode just by the nature of what we watched on the screen. Research has shown that simply looking at scenes of nature reduced heart rate, blood pressure and stress putting the body in the rest and restore state. Conversely, looking at or watching things that are scary, hearing about violence, watching people protest on the evening news or even enjoying a good adventure film, cause our bodies to naturally go into the fight or flight mode which results in an increase in heart rate, blood pressure and stress. A body in this mode can't rest and restore because it is getting the message that there is danger present, a response that helped primitive man survive, but today just results in difficulty sleeping.

Believe it or not, screens also affect our eating habits. When we are focusing our attention on a screen and not on our eating, we tend to eat more. This lack of attention causes us to miss the message our body sends out saying it's had enough. If we are engaged in something on the screen we are less mindful of our eating. We chew less and replace each mouthful in a robotic way. It's fairly typical of many people to consume less healthy snack type foods while watching television or a movie and they are amazed when they find they've eaten an entire package of whatever snack they were enjoying. Eating foods that offer minimal nutrition paired with eating larger amounts than necessary while engaging in a sedentary behavior can result in increased inflammation and weight gain.

Screen time impacts our relationships with others and the amount of time we spend fostering solid social connections, too. Screen time is often spent alone. You don't need others because the entertainment is on the screen. How often do you find yourself scrolling through social media when you could be interacting with your family or friends? If you are gathered with others around a screen the purpose is probably to watch a movie or sporting event and the expectation is that everyone is quiet and focused. This inhibits social interactions with the people sharing the experience. This is true of video games, also. Two children can be seated side by side playing a video game "together", however there is very little interaction between the two as they are focusing their attention on the game. The amount of time you spend engaged with electronic devices, is time not spent with others in your social network. Time that could be spent telling stories, playing games or finding out about each other's day is lost. Time gone by cannot be reclaimed. Children grow quickly, seasons fly by and months turn into years. Screens have the capacity to claim a lot of that time if we are not mindful.

When thinking about screen time in relation to your family, it is important to think about the time adults and children are spending on screens at work and at school, too. You know how much time you spend engaged with a screen while at work. It is important to also know that your school age children are also probably on computers regularly throughout the day. Much of their skill practice is through educational activities on the computer. Schools are purchasing site licenses in order to access quality, academically oriented online programs to support and complement their curricula. What used to be handwritten is now often done on the computer. Kids compose stories, write reports and do homework assignments on laptops instead of paper. This, too, is here to stay, but we must be mindful of this when we are determining how much screen time is healthy for our children. If you have school age children, you might give yourself the homework assignment of talking with your child's teacher to find out how much time is being spent in front of screens on an average day. Use this and the information in the next section to guide your screen limits at home.

The American Academy of Pediatrics (AAP) set forth new guidelines regarding children and media in October of 2016. They, too, recognize that children are growing up immersed in media, and caution parents to be mindful of how much media their children are exposed to each day. The AAP stresses that too much media use can be unhealthy and that parents must make sure their children have time to play, talk, do homework and sleep and state that, "Problems begin when media use displaces physical activity, hands-on exploration and face-to-face social interaction in the real world, which is critical to learning." They encourage "parents to be their child's 'media mentor'…… teaching them how to use it as a tool to create, connect and learn." Part of every parent's job is to guide their children in the choices they make and to educate them about the best ways to behave in various situations. This now includes making choices regarding screen time and teaching digital citizenship, or appropriate online behavior. Parents need to carefully monitor screen time and there should be clearly established limits regarding time spent on media, the types of media to which children have access (i.e. children's programming, video games, the internet and social media) and the content. To give parents a clearer idea of appropriate media interaction for children the AAP set forth suggested parameters. (See Suggested Media Time Recommendations chart on pages 83 and 84.)

Finally, AAP has also created a tool to help parents and caregivers create a personalized plan for media use based on the ages, needs and activities of their family called Create Your Family Media Plan. This user-friendly tool allows adults to plan for each child separately and incorporates time spent at school, eating, playing, doing homework, engaged in sports/practices, sleep and more. It is available at www.healthychildren.org, a website produced and managed by the American Academy of Pediatrics to guide and inform parents on current topics pertaining to parenting and child development.

Suggested Media Time Recommendations

Age	Media Time Recommendations	Other Recommendations
< 18 months	Avoid screen time	• Can expose to video chatting with family
18-24 months	No specific time recommended	• May expose to high quality programming • Watch with them and talk about what they are seeing
2-5 years of age	No more than an hour a day	• High quality programming • Parents should co-view to help with understanding and application to the world around them
6 and older	Place consistent limits on time spent on media	• Limit types of media • Make sure media time doesn't take the place of sleep, activity and other healthy behaviors

Suggested Media Time Recommendations (cont.)

Age	Media Time Recommendations	Other Recommendations
All children		<ul><li>Designate media free times (i.e. meal times, in the car)</li><li>Designate media free areas of the home (i.e. bedrooms, other unsupervised areas)</li><li>Computers should be located in main areas of the home for all to use</li></ul>

American Academy of Pediatrics 2016

You now have the knowledge needed to create a healthy schedule for your family. A well-balanced schedule accommodates the wellness needs of each family member. It provides the necessary structure and predictability to make each day flow with a sense of organization and calmness. It allows ample time for healthy eating, a variety of movement opportunities, time to connect and interact socially and time to relax and spend time doing what we really enjoy. It also incorporates regular sleep schedules that allow the body the time it needs to cleanse, repair and rejuvenate in preparation for another day. While the schedule may differ some from day to day, it should include rituals and routines around pivotal points in your family's day; getting up and ready in the morning, meals and bedtime. We are all creatures of habit and thrive best, body, mind and spirit, when we live with structure and predictability. Create a well-balanced schedule and enjoy a family life has less stress, more energy and happiness and better health.

Chapter Eleven

Taking Time for You

(A Message for Parents)

The best gift you can give your child is a healthy, happy you. Even the youngest infants sense and respond to stress. A baby will cry in the arms of an adult who feels nervous holding them or tending to their needs. Older children also sense and respond to a parent's stress or general stress in their environment, often becoming stressed and anxious themselves. When we, as parents, become stressed we are unable to effectively meet our own needs or the needs of others.

Life can seem like a juggling act with work and household responsibilities along with parenting. A life comprised of moving from one responsibility to the next with no time to slow down, is not a life responsibly lived. You may feel it is necessary in the moment, and that there's no other way to accomplish the things that need doing, however, as time goes by you'll become less able to manage the day to day responsibilities well. You can only keep the wheels turning at a fast pace for so long. In order to be the productive person you want to be and the responsible parent that your children deserve, you need to give yourself the gift of some unstructured time each day. Your body and brain need time to relax. Leaving room in the schedule for you to slow down is imperative. You need and deserve time to connect with loved ones in meaningful ways, to engage in activities you enjoy and to practice some self-care. When did you last read a book, take a warm bath, go for a walk all by yourself or just relax with a friend and enjoy a coffee or tea. These are the things that allow us to find relaxation and joy in our day. These are the very things that make life worth living. Loving and taking care of yourself, enable you to love and take care of those who rely on you in the best possible way.

Adults need unstructured time as much as kids do. It's imperative that you find time each day, even if it's just a bit, to rest, relax and pamper yourself. It might mean getting the kids to bed a bit earlier, so you have time to read your favorite magazine, or watch your favorite show uninterrupted. It might mean stopping at the gym on your way home from work and paying a few extra dollars for daycare. It might mean getting up a half hour earlier to start your day with a hot cup of coffee to drink as you just sit and enjoy the sunrise. Find whatever is relaxing and enjoyable to you and make it part of your day.

Practicing self-care and feeling good about yourself, the way you look and the way you feel are key to being able to deliver well on the day to day responsibilities. Feeling good about yourself can make all the difference in the outcome of your day. Be sure that you make time to shower, shave, do your hair and put on a presentable outfit that makes you feel good. Even if you're the parent of a colicky infant, taking the time for self-care will make you better able to manage the day ahead of you and care for your baby. Clothes that are clean and fit well will set you up for a more positive day than a pair of baggy sweatpants and a t-shirt you wore the evening before. Even if you're not planning on leaving the house, get yourself cleaned up and ready to face the day in a positive way. What we wear and our perception of how we look actually affect our mood, self-esteem and output. It can be summed up in the phrase dress for success.

As parents we spend a lot of time with our children no matter what their age. We care for and nurture them, play with them, teach them and support them as they venture out and try new things. We are responsible for their health and welfare. We are bonded with our children in a different way than we will ever be connected with another person, yet we need to make sure that in addition to spending time with them and taking time for ourselves we also nourish our adult relationships.

Spending unstructured time with other adults lets us enjoy being a grown-up for a while and allows us to step out of our role as a parent. Spending time with friends or our partner or spouse in a relaxed atmosphere gives us the opportunity to talk about and do adult things. It allows us to connect with and enjoy important people in our lives. Solid social connections are crucial to your overall health. Research has indicated that solid social connections are one of the common markers for longevity and freedom from chronic disease around the world.

When we take time out to nurture our adult relationships we improve our parenting, too. Remember the phrase, absence makes the heart grow fonder. We can apply this to parenthood. As much as we love our children and enjoy being with them, time apart is healthy and warranted for both parents and children. Every parent has those days when they feel they can't handle one more tear, one more tantrum or one more argument. It's good for even the youngest of children to realize that others can care for them and that you will return. If you don't have family nearby, it's important to make connections with people in your neighborhood or community, so that you have others available to help with child care giving you the time you need to reboot. You'll return home feeling refreshed and ready to take on the next adventure.

If you have a spouse or partner, taking the time to nurture your relationship is crucial. It's easy to get wrapped up in the day to day routine; working, taking care of the kids, making the meals and tidying up after everyone, and never really connect with that important person in your life. Even if you are both tired at the end of the day it's important to find at least a few minutes to talk or share some time together. Parenting is demanding and tiring, and it's easy to fall into these habits and unknowingly neglect your relationship with your significant other. After all, you see them every day. They are a constant in your life. Hopefully, you have a solid relationship and are there for each other no matter what the circumstance. In a good relationship your partner is integral to your happiness. Nourishing this relationship is as important as caring for and nourishing your children. Make sure you build in time for just the two of you. Try to connect in some way every day. It can be right at home after the kids are in bed, or it may be a night out. Schedule times to spend together. Put them on the calendar. Maybe even call them Date Nights. Planned outings with your partner give you both something to look forward to, as well as provide opportunities to nurture your relationship. They give you the time you need to reconnect and enjoy each other, time to recharge your spirits and relationship, time to talk about your wants and desires and time to dream about your future together.

Take the time to nourish your body and soul on a regular basis. Everyone will benefit. Your children will learn the importance of self-nurture through your example, as well as discover that they can get along without you for periods of time. You will relax, renew and be able to enjoy some of life's simple pleasures in the company of other adults and by yourself which will, in turn, make you a better parent.

Final Thoughts

In closing, remember the human body is an amazing machine that can withstand and adapt to many conditions. If not well cared for, the body weakens and chronic disease sets in. Given the time to relax and renew daily, given a good quality diet and plenty of movement and given the chance to cleanse and rejuvenate every night your body will take you far. Take care not to push it too much. Unlike so many other things in life, it is not replaceable. It's your job to treat it with care and compassion and to know when to put the brakes on. And for the too few years you are entrusted with the lives of your children and their welfare, it is your job to take exemplary care of their bodies, also. You now have the tools to do that. Make it your priority to find a healthy balance and nurture them; body, mind and spirit.

As parents, we have two important roles in our children's lives; to give them roots and wings. By choosing to make positive lifestyle changes within your family you are giving your children solid roots. When it comes time for them to use their wings, they will fly away equipped with the tools to live a life of abundant health.

Enjoy your journey!

References

"5 Omega-Rich Seeds You Should Include in Your Daily Diet." EcoWatch. N. p. n. d. Web. Feb. 2018.

Allais, L., Boon, N. Bracke, K. R., Brusselle, G. G., Cuvelier, C.A., De Smet, R., Kerckhof, F. M., Laukens, D., Van den, Abbeele P., De Vos, M., Van de Wiele, T. and Verschuere, S. "Chronic cigarette smoke exposure induces microbial and inflammatory shifts and mucin changes in the murine gut". National Center for Biotechnology Information, US National Library of Medicine. n. d. Web. Feb. 2018.

"American Academy of Pediatrics Announces New Recommendations for Children's Media Use". American Academy of Pediatrics. N. p. n. d. Web. March 2018.

"Anti-bacterial cleaning products". Better Health Channel. State Government of Victoria Australia. Dept. of Health and Human Services. May 2017. Web. Feb. 2018.

Axe, Dr. Josh. Eat Dirt; Why Leaky Gut May Be the Root Cause of your Health Problems and 5 Surprising Steps to Cure it. New York. HarperCollins. 2016. 59-60. Print.

Bird, Anthony and Conlon, Michael. "The Impact of Diet and Lifestyle on Gut Microbiota and Human Health". Nutrients. National Center for Biotechnology Information, US National Library of Medicine. n. d. Web. Feb. 2018.

"Blue Light Has A Dark Side". Harvard Health Publishing, Harvard Medical School. Harvard University. 30 Dec. 2017. Web. March 2018.

"Colds in Children". National Center for Biotechnology Information, US National Library of Medicine, n. d. Web. Feb. 2018.

"Differences Between Organics and Conventionally Grown Foods". Food Safety and You.com. Center for Food Service Learning, LLC. n.d. Web. Jan. 2018.

Engen P.A., Green S.J, Voigt R.M., Forsyth T.B. and Keshavarzian A. "The Gastrointestinal Microbiome: Alcohol Effects on the Composition of the Intestinal Microbiota". **National Center for Biotechnology Information, US National Library of Medicine. n. d. Web. Feb. 2018.**

Environmental Working Group. EWG. N. p. n.d. Web. Jan. 2018.

"Exercise for Your Bone Health". National Institutes of Health. Osteoporosis and Related Bone Diseases National Resource Center, n.d. Web. March 2018.

Ferguson, J. L. "How Clothing Choices Affect and Reflect Your Self-Image". HuffPost. N. p. 5 Feb. 2017. Web. March 2018.

Fields, H. The Gut: Where Bacteria and Immune System Meet. The Johns Hopkins University. n. d. Web. Feb. 2018.

"Foods to Restore Your Intestinal Flora". Scientific American. Springer Nature. n.d. Web. Feb. 2018.

Francino, M.P. "Antibiotics and the Human Gut Microbiome: Disbioses and Accumulation of Resistances". **National Center for Biotechnology Information, US National Library of Medicine. n. d. Web. Feb. 2018.**

"Global Strategy on Diet, Physical Activity and Health". World Health Organization. N. p. n.d. Web. Jan. 2018.

Griffiths, C and Santor, J with Goodall, D. "Free Play in Early Childhood; A literature review". Play England. National Children's Bureau. n.d. Web. March 2018.

"Growing up with a pet may boot a baby's bacterial health". National Center for Biotechnology Information, US National Library of Medicine. Pub Med Health. n. d. Web. Feb. 2018.

"How Does the Immune System Work?" National Center for Biotechnology Information, US National Library of Medicine. Pub Med Health. 21 Sept. 2016. Web. Feb. 2018.

"How to Make a Family Media Use Plan". healthy children.org. Powered by pediatricians. Trusted by parents. American Academy of Pediatrics. n. d. Web. March 2018.

Jockers. David M.D. "The Top 33 Prebiotic Foods for Your Digestive System". Dr. Jockers.com. Supercharge Your Health. N. p. n.d. Web. Feb. 2018.

Macdonald, Fiona. "Antibacterial Ingredient Can Really Quickly Mess with Gut Bacteria, Study Finds". Science Alert. N. p. n.d. Web. Jan 2018.

Mercola, Joseph M.D. "Research Reveals the Importance of Your Microbiome for Optimal Health". Mercola. N. p. n.d. Web. Feb. 2018.

Mercola, Joseph M.D. "Should 15,000 Steps A Day Be Your New Goal?" Fitness Peak. Mercola. n. d. Web. March 2018.

"My Plate". Wikipedia. Wikimedia Foundation, Inc. N. p. 9 Feb. 2018. Web. Jan. 2018.

Neu, Josef, MD and Rushing, Jona, MD. "Cesarean versus Vaginal Delivery: Long term infant outcomes and the Hygiene Hypothesis. National Center for Biotechnology Information, US National Library of Medicine. n. d. Web. Feb. 2018.

"Pesticides and Food: Healthy, Sensible Food Practices". United States Environmental Protection Agency. United States Government. 19 Jan. 2017. Web. Jan. 2018.

"Price Look Up Codes". International Federation for Produce Standards. N. p. n.d. Web. Jan. 2018.

"Probiotics: In Depth". National Center for Complementary and Integrative Health. United States. Dept. of Health and Human Services. n.d. Web. Feb. 2018.

The Pubic Health and Safety Organization. NSF. N. p. n.d. Web. Jan. 2018.

"Short-Term Effect of Antibiotics on Human Gut Microbiota". National Center for Biotechnology Information, US National Library of Medicine. n. d. Web. Feb. 2018.

"The 4 Happy Hormones". Joyful Days. Live well. Be happy. N. p. n.d. Web. March 2018.

"The Brain-Gut Connection". Johns Hopkins Medicine. Johns Hopkins University. n.d. Web. Feb. 2018.

United States Department of Agriculture. ChooseMyPlate.gov. US Department of Agriculture. 7 Dec. 2016. Web. Jan. 2018.

"What Does Organic Mean? Organic.org N. p. n.d. Web. Jan. 2018.

"What Is GMO". The Non-GMO Project. N. p. 14 Feb. 2018. Web. Jan. 2018.

"Where Did Agriculture Begin? Oh Boy, It's Complicated". The Salt. What's On Your Plate. NPR. n.d. Web. Jan 2018.

"Why is physical activity so important for health and wellbeing?". American Heart Association. N. p. 14. Dec. 2016. Web. March 2018.

Wilson, Ian and Nicholson, Jeremy. "Gut Microbiome Interactions with Drug Metabolism, Efficacy and Toxicity". **National Center for Biotechnology Information, US National Library of Medicine. n. d. Web. Feb. 2018.**

9 781717 521217